Common Breast Lesions

Generously illustrated with more than 650 photographs, drawings, histopathology slides, radiographs, and mammograms, this color atlas provides a step-by-step guide to the differential diagnosis and treatment of the most prevalent cancerous and noncancerous breast diseases. Written by a multidisciplinary team of specialists, Part One focuses on benign tumors, malignant neoplasms, pain, and various symptoms of the skin and nipple-areola complex. Part Two provides a guide to proper clinical examination; diagnostic and interventional radiology; diagnostic pathology; surgical biopsy; surgical excision of benign lesions; breast conservation surgery; excision of the sentinel node; total, modified, and radical mastec-

tomies; and reconstructive surgery. Primary care physicians will find this guide invaluable for diagnosing, referring, and educating patients. Specialists will appreciate the practical tips and illustrated techniques for treating the most common cancers affecting women today.

Dr. Samuel Pilnik is Attending Breast Surgeon at Lenox Hill Hospital in New York City and Associate Professor of Surgery at New York Medical College. His practice is devoted to surgical breast oncology. Over the course of his career, this Fellow of the American College of Surgeons and the International College of Surgeons has treated more than 14,000 patients with breast disease.

Common Breast Lesions

A Photographic Guide to Diagnosis and Treatment

Edited by

SAMUEL PILNIK

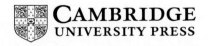
CAMBRIDGE
UNIVERSITY PRESS

PUBLISHED BY THE PRESS SYNDICATE OF THE UNIVERSITY OF CAMBRIDGE
The Pitt Building, Trumpington Street, Cambridge, United Kingdom

CAMBRIDGE UNIVERSITY PRESS
The Edinburgh Building, Cambridge CB2 2RU, UK
40 West 20th Street, New York, NY 10011-4211, USA
477 Williamstown Road, Port Melbourne, VIC 3207, Australia
Ruiz de Alarcón 13, 28014 Madrid, Spain
Dock House, The Waterfront, Cape Town 8001, South Africa

http://www.cambridge.org

First published 2003

Printed in Singapore

Typeface Stone Serif 9.5/13 pts.   *System* QuarkXPress™   [HT]

A catalog record for this book is available from the British Library

Library of Congress Cataloging-in-Publication Data

Common breast lesions : a photographic guide to diagnosis and
treatment / edited by Samuel Pilnik.
      p. ; cm.
   Includes bibliographical references and index.
   ISBN 0-521-82357-9 (hardback)
     1. Breast—Cancer—Atlases. 2. Breast—Diseases—Atlases.
I. Pilnik, Samuel, 1929–
   [DNLM: 1. Breast Diseases—diagnosis—Atlases. 2. Breast
Diseases—therapy—Atlases.
  WP 17 C734 2003]
  RC280.B8 C623 2003
  618.1'9'0222—dc21   2002191146

Every effort has been made in preparing this book to provide
accurate and up-to-date information that is in accord with accepted
standards and practice at the time of publication. Nevertheless, the
authors, editors, and publisher can make no warranties that the
information contained herein is totally free from error, not least
because clinical standards are constantly changing through research
and regulation. The authors, editors, and publisher therefore disclaim
all liability for direct or consequential damages resulting from the
use of material contained in this book. Readers are strongly advised
to pay careful attention to information provided by the manufacturer
of any drugs or equipment that they plan to use.

Contributing Authors

EDITOR

Samuel Pilnik, MD
Attending Breast Surgeon
Lenox Hill Hospital
Clinical Associate Professor of Surgery
New York Medical College
New York, New York

CONTRIBUTING AUTHORS

Susan Jormark, MD
Attending Pathologist
Lenox Hill Hospital
Clinical Assistant Professor of Pathology
New York University
New York, New York

Evan Morton, MD
Attending Radiologist
Section Chief of Women Imaging
Lenox Hill Hospital
New York, New York

Fred Pezzulli, MD
Attending Radiologist
Assistant Chief, Breast Imaging
Lenox Hill Hospital
New York, New York

Norman H. Schulman, MD
Attending Surgeon
Director, Division of Plastic and Reconstructive
    Surgery
Lenox Hill Hospital
New York, New York

To my wife with gratitude for her quiet faith and the contagious sympathy she has demonstrated during my entire medical career.

A breast lump in a woman should be considered
malignant until it is proven it is not.

— Bloodgood

Contents

Preface

This book is intended to be a basic guide in the diagnosis and surgical treatment of breast lesions. The goal was to produce a book that would not only be suited to the needs of medical students, but also one that the student would carry into practice. It represents the crystallization of my personal experience based on 14,000 records of patients with diseases of the breast that I have treated during the last 35 years. Throughout all these years, I have continuously photographed patients with demonstrable and visible clinical problems. I have used this material for the purpose of teaching medical students, residents, and physicians involved in the care of female patients. As they have found my photographic library of enormous benefit as a reference guide, I decided to write this textbook in the form of an atlas.

I believe that a guideline should be simple and practical. With this in mind, only the most common breast lesions seen in daily practice are discussed. The reader is referred to the many textbooks available for the more complex and rare breast lesions. A list of suggested readings is provided at the end of this text. Traditional basic science chapters on anatomy, embryology, and physiology were purposely omitted. When appropriate, basic science is discussed in the pertinent clinical sections. Some mammogram images and histopathology are included in the discussion of each clinical problem, leading to some inevitable duplication. Throughout my years of teaching I have learned that this format is the most practical.

The diagnosis and surgical management of breast diseases are now multidisciplinary. This was not so 30 years ago when, besides the clinical examination, the only diagnostic procedures consisted of a mammogram and the pathology diagnosis after the lesions were excised or a mastectomy performed. I have had the rare opportunity to witness the progress in diagnosis and surgical treatment that has occurred. The multidisciplinary approach requires the combined efforts of the clinician, the radiologist, the pathologist, and the surgeon. This textbook is organized to reflect a multidisciplinary approach.

The clinician's care of the female patient is the initial challenge. The clinician should not only know the clinical presentation and the clinical differential diagnosis of the most common breast lesions but also should be able to thoroughly and systematically examine the patient. The role of the radiologist in this multidisciplinary approach has changed over time. It is no longer limited to the imaging of the breast but often includes aiding the clinician and the surgeon when making a diagnosis with noninvasive procedures such as a core biopsy under ultrasound or stereotactic techniques. The radiologist also plays a role in assisting the surgeon to accurately remove nonpalpable lesions by guided imaging.

In the mid-twenties, Bloodgood stated that "every surgeon should be his own pathologist." This is no longer possible today. The pathologist's role is not only to interpret the frozen and permanent tissue section but also to inform the surgeon of the breast cancer markers so the most appropriate cancer care treatments are chosen. Before the mid-seventies the treatment of breast cancer was limited to radical mastectomy with or without radiation therapy. Currently because breast cancer is diagnosed at an earlier stage, less radical procedures to the breast and the axilla are now available. Because of the scope of this book, only the technical aspects of treatment will be discussed. The availability and progress made in the reconstruction of the breast provides the patient with some comfort to her physical changes and the psychological impact that breast cancer causes. A section on breast reconstruction is included to serve as a guide to the clinician and the surgeon in counseling their patients.

For many years I have had the privilege to closely work with Doctors Susan Jormark, Evan Morton, Fred

Pezzulli, and Norman Schulman. I would like to express to them my indebtedness for their expert contributions and for their immediate understanding of the purpose of this book. I am very grateful to Doctor Olga Tsireshkin for providing the MRI illustrations for the section "The Role of the Radiologist." I would like to also express my enduring gratitude to my patients for their courtesy and willingness to allow me to photograph them over the years for the express purpose of imparting valuable information to others. I have learned much of what I have written from them. I would also like to thank Mr. George Tanis and Ms. Sophie Benarz for the photographic skills they have displayed in both the operating room and the photography studio. Finally, I would like to pass on my appreciation to Cambridge University Press for undertaking this publication and to my editor, Ms. Heidi Lovette, for her expert direction.

Reasons for Breast Consultation

1

Benign Tumors

A tumor in the breast is the most common complaint for which a woman consults a physician. Patients refer to this finding as a "lump," "thickening," or "mass." The physician oftentimes also uses that terminology. But because "mass" and "tumor" have different clinical significance, the physician should be able to distinguish between them.

Figures 1.1 and 1.2

A tumor is a clinical entity that has three dimensions: width, height, and depth.

For didactic purposes, a tumor can be compared with a rubber ball (Figure 1.1). With the rubber ball held hidden halfway within the palm of one hand, the protruding surface of the ball is palpated using the index and second fingers of the opposite hand. Because of the perception of depth ("stereognosis"), the clinician (or the patient during self-examination) can perceive that there is "something behind" that surface (Figure 1.2).

On the other hand, a mass is an entity that has only two dimensions: width and length. On examination, the clinician can feel an area of thickening that, at each extreme, blends with the breast tissue rather than forming a defined edge. A mass is a clin-

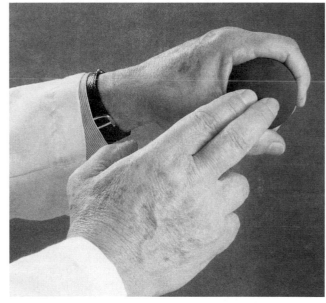

FIGURE 1.2

ical finding present in some histologic types of fibrocystic changes, such as hyperplasia (see "Fibrocystic Changes" later in this chapter).

Approximately 70% of breast tumors are benign. The fact that 30% of all breast lesions could be malignant is significant. The physician should not only be aware of these percentages but should also know which breast lesions are the most common and how to make a clinical differential diagnosis.

The breast problems most commonly seen in a medical practice not specialized in breast diseases are fibroadenoma and some of its variants – giant fibroadenoma, juvenile fibroadenoma, and hamartoma – and phyllodes tumors, cysts, and cancers. Because this textbook is intended as a guide for physicians and general surgeons whose practices include the care of women, only the most common breast tumors and their surgical treatment are discussed. For less common tumors, the reader is referred to the textbooks and literature listed in "Suggested Readings" at the back of this book.

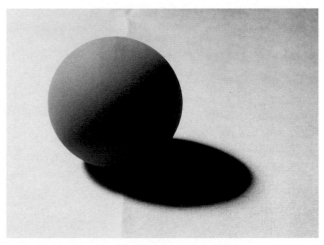

FIGURE 1.1

FIBROADENOMA

After fibrocystic changes, fibroadenomas are the most common benign breast lesion, with an incidence of 18%–20%. Fibroadenomas are found accidentally during breast self-examination or during routine clinical breast examination, mammography, or ultrasonography.

CLINICAL PRESENTATION

Fibroadenomas are usually asymptomatic. However, in cases in which an intratumoral hemorrhage has occurred, pain could be the initial presenting symptom. Such a presentation is more common in pregnant or lactating women.

In general, fibroadenomas present as a single tumor, varying in size from 1 cm to 4 cm. Multiple tumors are found in about 10%–12% of cases, and they can occur either simultaneously or metachronously.

The causes of fibroadenoma are unknown; but because fibroadenomas do not occur before menarche, a relationship to ovarian secretion of estrogen is considered likely. The age incidence is 20–30 years, with a peak incidence in women just over the age of 30.

Fibroadenomas do not change in size during the menstrual cycle, but a preexisting fibroadenoma may increase in size during pregnancy.

Fibroadenoma rarely occurs late in life. When the tumor is diagnosed in older patients, it most likely has been present from a younger age and been undetected. In elderly patients, fibroadenomas may undergo involutional change. This degenerative change is due either to increased stromal growth or to an unrecognized infarction with necrosis. The result is calcification or a hyalinized fibroadenoma. Calcified fibroadenomas, especially of the lobulated type (called "popcorn" lesions), may be mistaken on physical examination for carcinomas. The difference is that a calcified fibroadenoma retains its mobility.

For the most part, fibroadenomas are benign tumors. The malignant potential of a fibroadenoma is very low, the incidence being in the range of 3 in 1000 cases.

Because fibroadenomas develop from the lobule, lobular carcinoma is the most common of cancer found within a fibroadenoma. Ductal carcinoma in situ has also been reported. The clinical behavior of carcinoma arising within a fibroadenoma is probably equivalent to that of malignant tumors arising elsewhere in the breast. Malignancy in a fibroadenoma is usually an incidental finding.

PHYSICAL EXAMINATION

The characteristics of a fibroadenoma depend on the relationship between its two main histologic components, the acinar epithelium and the connective tissue. The examiner should record delineation, consistency, presence or absence of tenderness on palpation, and mobility.

Figures 1.3 and 1.4

When epithelial proliferation is the main component of a fibroadenoma, the surface of the tumor is smooth. The gross specimen of a fibroadenoma in Figure 1.3 shows the smooth, oval or round surface

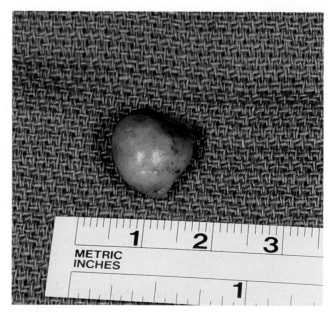

FIGURE 1.3

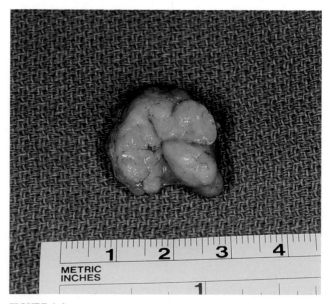

FIGURE 1.4

felt in a clinical examination. When the epithelial component of a fibroadenoma is compressed within preponderant connective tissue, the surface of the tumor becomes lobulated (Figure 1.4). In either case, the fibroadenoma has an ovoid or spherical shape, is mobile, and is non-tender to palpation.

Figures 1.5 and 1.6

Fibroadenomas are well-delineated tumors with smooth margins. The delineation (as well as the smoothness and consistency) is best appreciated by supporting the tumor with the index finger and thumb of the non-dominant hand and then feeling the surface of the tumor with the index finger of the

dominant hand (Figure 1.5). The surface of a fibroadenoma is usually uniformly smooth (Figure 1.6). However if a large amount of fibrous tissue encircles the epithelial elements, the glandular portion between the fibrous tissue will be compressed and will bulge, causing a lobulated surface (Figure 1.4).

Figures 1.7 and 1.8

The consistency of a fibroadenoma is "rubbery". It is described as such because of the similarity with the consistency of a rubber ball (Figure 1.7). The consistency may also be similar to the cartilaginous consistency of the tip of the nose (Figure 1.8).

Fibroadenomas are not tender on palpation.

Figures 1.9 and 1.10

Another physical characteristic of a fibroadenoma is its mobility. This mobility can be elicited by pressing on one side of the tumor with one finger (Figure 1.9). The tumor moves away from the finger with a "bounce back" motion when the finger is released. The mobility of the lesion is explained by

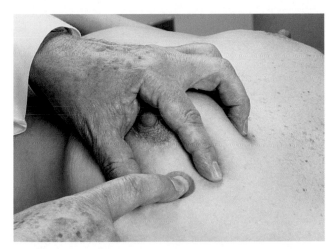

FIGURE 1.5

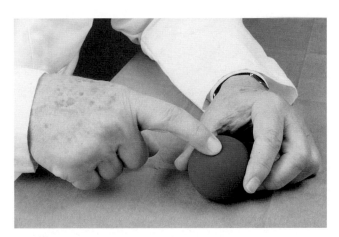

FIGURE 1.7

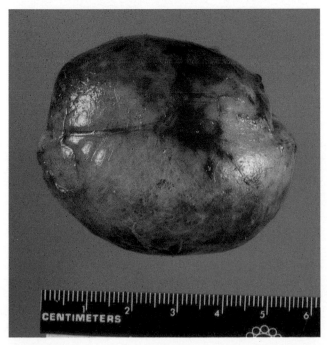

FIGURE 1.6

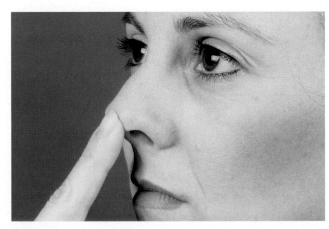

FIGURE 1.8

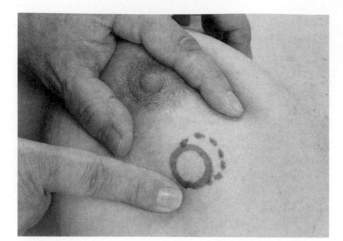

FIGURE 1.9

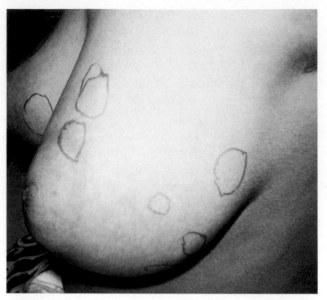

FIGURE 1.11

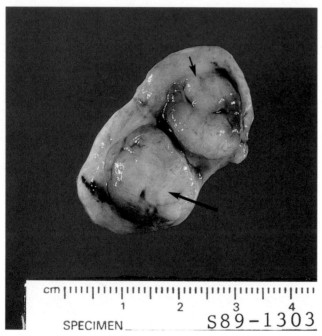

FIGURE 1.10

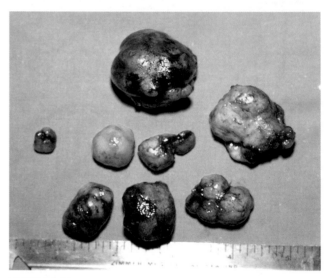

FIGURE 1.12

its structure. Fibroadenomas are separated from the surrounding breast tissue by a thin, loose layer of connective tissue often called a "capsule." (See chapter 9, The Role of the Pathologist, Figure 9.28.)

The gross specimen of a fibroadenoma in Figure 1.10 was bisected to demonstrate the sharp delineation between the tumor and the rim of normal tissue that was excised with the lesion (small arrow). The bulging cut surface is also characteristic of a fibroadenoma (large arrow).

Figures 1.11 and 1.12

Fibroadenomas can be multiple and bilateral. The incidence of multiple or bilateral fibroadenoma

is approximately 10%–12%. Figure 1.11 shows a 21-year-old patient with bilateral synchronous multiple fibroadenomas. Ten were found on the left breast and eight on the right breast. Figure 1.12 shows the specimens excised from the right breast. All have the typical gross characteristic of a fibroadenoma – that is, a well delineated and glistening surface.

IMAGING

In patients aged 20–30 years (the age group in which fibroadenoma is the most common lesion), mammography has a poor diagnostic yield. Ultrasonography not only spares the radiation, it also has a better yield to demonstrate the lesion.

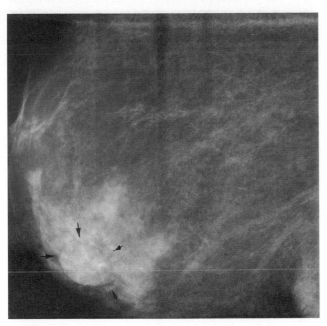

FIGURE 1.13

Figure 1.13

On mammography, a fibroadenoma images as a well-delineated tumor with sharp margins. Sometimes the mammogram will also image a thin, lucent line called a "halo" surrounding the tumor. The halo represents the connective tissue that separates the fibroadenoma from the surrounding breast tissue.

The mammogram in Figure 1.13 shows the smooth, marginated mass of a fibroadenoma 1.2 cm × 2 cm located in the retroareolar region of the breast. Note the lucent "halo" surrounding the mass, suggesting a benign entity (arrows).

Figure 1.14

On ultrasonography, a fibroadenoma is sharply circumscribed with an oval or round shape, an internal echo pattern (A), and posterior acoustic shadowing (B) (see chapter 8, "Role of the Radiologist").

Figures 1.15 and 1.16

The image pattern of a calcified fibroadenoma depends on the stromal elements that the tumor contains. When the fibroadenoma is uniformly cellular, the calcification will be smooth. Figure 1.15 shows a mammogram of a partially calcified fibroadenoma within a soft tissue mass (arrow). The

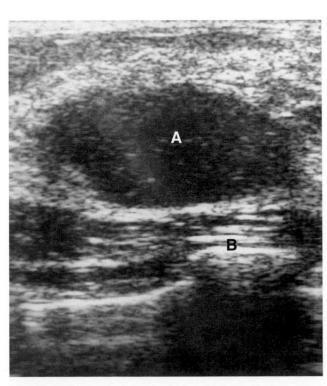

FIGURE 1.14

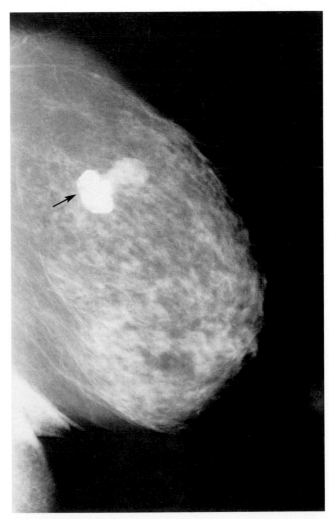

FIGURE 1.15

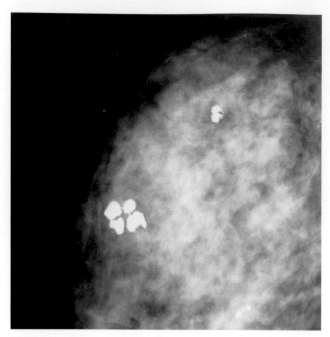

FIGURE 1.16

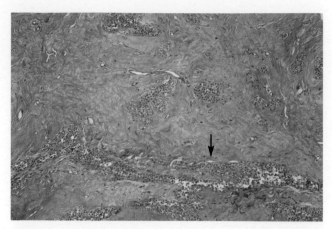

FIGURE 1.17

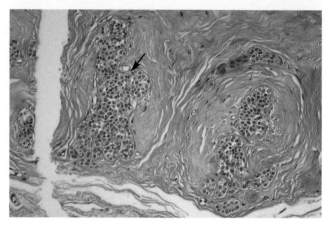

FIGURE 1.18

tumor is predominantly cellular, similar to the one shown in Figure 1.3. The calcification is smooth.

In fibroadenomas in which the fibrous elements predominate and encircle the epithelial elements, the calcification images on the mammogram with a characteristic "popcorn" appearance. The mammogram in Figure 1.16 shows a lobulated fibroadenoma with dystrophic calcifications (similar to the fibroadenoma shown in Figure 1.4).]

TREATMENT

Treatment for fibroadenoma is surgical. These tumors are the most commonly excised benign solid breast lesions. Excision of single and multiple fibroadenomas is discussed in chapter 11, "Surgical Treatment of Benign Breast Lesions." When malignancy is present within a fibroadenoma (Figures 1.17 and 1.18), the treatment options are the same as those applied to similar malignant lesions not associated with fibroadenoma.

Figure 1.17
Figure 1.17 shows a low-power light microscopy view of a fibroadenoma that developed lobular carcinoma in situ. The ducts are distended and hypercellular (arrow).

Figure 1.18
Figure 1.18 shows a higher-power light microscopy view of the fibroadenoma in Figure 1.17.

Notice that the cells are arranged in the typical pattern of lobular carcinoma: monomorphic cells with uniform, dark nuclei and scant cytoplasm (arrow).

FIBROADENOMA VARIANTS

Giant Fibroadenoma

A giant fibroadenoma is a fibroadenoma larger than 5 cm. It is not usual for a giant fibroadenoma to reach a size of 8–10 cm, the average size being 5–10 cm. Cases of giant fibroadenomas weighing 500 g have been reported, but such occurrences are rare.

CLINICAL PRESENTATION

The age incidence for giant fibroadenoma has two peaks: adolescence and perimenopause. Characteristically, giant fibroadenomas of adolescence (Figure 1.19) grow suddenly and may be mistaken for rapid normal breast development. The sudden enlargement is usually accompanied by pain.

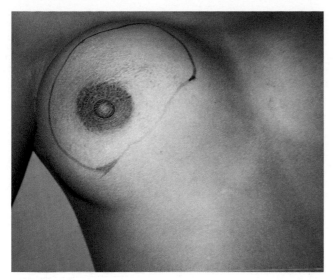

FIGURE 1.19

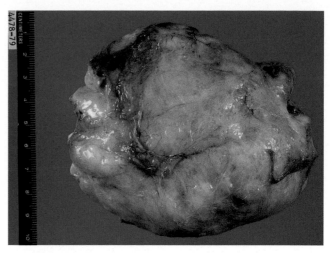

FIGURE 1.20

This mastodynia is non-cyclical, being due to the space that the tumor occupies within the breast. Giant fibroadenomas of perimenopause present a differential diagnosis challenge in the clinic because they resemble phyllodes tumors in size.

Figure 1.19

Figure 1.19 shows giant fibroadenoma in a 16-year-old patient (enlarged right breast). Physical examination demonstrated asymmetry. No skin or nipple changes were present. The tumor was located in the retroareolar area and extended to both upper quadrants of the breast. The tumor measured 6 cm in diameter, was well marginated, had a smooth surface, and was mobile. The consistency was firm.

PHYSICAL EXAMINATION

On physical examination, giant fibroadenomas of adolescence and perimenopause are both firm in consistency. Both have well-defined borders. These clinical findings differentiate giant fibroadenomas from hypertrophy, a condition in which the breast enlarges and the parenchyma is diffusely firm at the expense of hypertrophy of the fibrous tissue. Breast hypertrophy lacks the defined borders of a giant fibroadenoma. A phyllodes tumor has a lobulated surface (see "Phyllodes Tumor" later in this subsection).

Figure 1.20

Figure 1.20 shows a gross specimen of giant fibroadenoma. Like all fibroadenomas, giant fibroadenomas are well encapsulated, but they are more "meaty" in consistency. Often, the gross appearance may resemble that of a phyllodes tumor; the difference is that the phyllodes tumors are not as well encapsulated.

IMAGING

Except for size, giant fibroadenomas image like fibroadenomas on mammography and ultrasound examination. The microscopic appearance is also similar to that of ordinary fibroadenomas.

TREATMENT

The management of giant fibroadenomas is surgical; they are excised for cosmetic reasons. As with ordinary fibroadenomas, simple excision is the treatment of choice. A core biopsy should be carried out preoperatively to confirm the diagnosis.

Being encapsulated tumors, giant fibroadenomas can – unlike phyllodes tumors – be excised using enucleation alone (Figure 1.20). Recurrence is not a concern.

Because of the size of the tumor, a frontal scar will inevitably leave an undesirable cosmetic result. Giant fibroadenomas should be excised using an incision along the lateral crease of the breast – the Gaillard–Thomas incision. (See "Excision of Multiple and Large Benign Tumors" in chapter 11, "Surgical Treatment of Benign Breast Lesions.")

Juvenile Fibroadenoma

Juvenile fibroadenoma is also a tumor of adolescence. Compared with fibroadenomas, juvenile fibroadenomas occur in younger patients and grow more rapidly.

PHYSICAL EXAMINATION

On physical examination, the tumor is not as well defined as an ordinary fibroadenoma. The consistency of the tumor is firm.

Figure 1.21

Microscopically, juvenile fibroadenomas have a more florid glandular hyperplasia and a greater stromal cellularity. The clinical significance of these traits is not well determined by pathologists.

Lipoma

The breast is composed of glandular tissue, fibrous tissue, and fat. It is therefore not surprising that a lipoma is occasionally diagnosed in the breast; however, a lipoma is not a primary tumor of the breast. Large lipomas usually originate from the interpectoral fat and protrude through the fibers of the pectoralis major muscle.

PHYSICAL EXAMINATION

The origin of a large lipoma can be proved during the physical examination by having the patient press both hands to her hips during the inspection. With this maneuver, the pectoralis major muscle contracts, and the lipoma protrudes through the muscle fibers. (See Figure 1.39 and 1.40 later in this chapter.)

Small lipomas of the breast can be missed on physical examination. The surface of the tumor is smooth, and its consistency is soft.

TREATMENT

Lipoma of the breast requires no treatment. Large lipomas – like the one shown in Figure 1.39 in

the discussion of phyllodes tumor – are removed for cosmesis.

Hamartoma

Hamartomas are benign breast tumors that contain fibroglandular and adipose tissue. For that reason, hamartomas have received various names such as "fibroadenolipoma," "adenolipoma," "lipofibroadenoma," and "adenofibroma."

CLINICAL PRESENTATION

Hamartomas are soft tumors that often resemble breast tissue in texture. They are asymptomatic and difficult to detect on physical examination. As a result, they are often found during routine mammography or ultrasonography examination.

The age incidence for hamartoma ranges between 18 years and 85 years, with a mean of 45–55 years (perimenopause and menopause).

PHYSICAL EXAMINATION

Hamartomas are spherical, well-delineated tumors with a smooth and uniform surface. Their consistency depends on the ratio between the fibroglandular tissue and the fat that they contain. When fatty tissue predominates, the lesion is soft and may resemble a lipoma. If fibroglandular tissue is more abundant, the hamartoma may have a firm consistency similar to a fibroadenoma. When fat is the main component of the tumor, a hamartoma may be missed on physical examination.

IMAGING

The mammographic image of a hamartoma is inconsistent. It varies depending on the proportion of fibroglandular tissue and fat present. Detection depends on the content of the particular tumor. Because fat is radiolucent, the lesion may go undiagnosed radiographically.

On ultrasound examination, hamartomas image as hypoechoic, nonhomogenous entities.

Figure 1.22

The mediolateral oblique (MLO) mammographic view of a hamartoma in Figure 1.22 demonstrates a well-circumscribed mass in the lower portion of the breast. The well-encapsulated mass (arrow) contains a mixture of solid and fatty components, producing a mottled pattern described as a "slice of sausage" appearance (arrow).

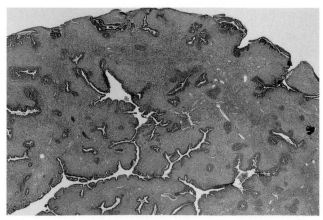

FIGURE 1.21

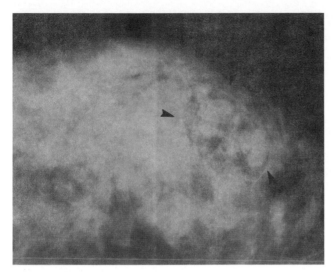

FIGURE 1.22

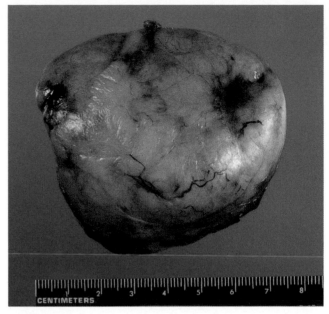

FIGURE 1.24

PATHOLOGY

Hamartomas are sharply circumscribed ovoid or spherical tumors. On gross examination, the color and consistency vary depending on the relative proportions of fat and epithelial and fibrous tissue (Figure 1.23). The color can vary from yellow to whitish yellow, and the consistency, from soft to firm. A fine-needle aspiration biopsy may be misrepresentative when the needle obtains only the fatty content of the tumor.

Figures 1.23 and 1.24

The gross specimen of a hamartoma in Figure 1.23 is well circumscribed, with a glistening, smooth surface and an ovoid shape. Its yellow color is due to its proportionately large fat component. A gross specimen of a fibroadenoma (Figure 1.24) is shown for differential diagnosis. Fibroadenomas are also ovoid, with a glistening surface and good demarcation, but their color is pinkish white, and their consistency is firm and rubbery.

Figure 1.25

This mounted gross section of a hamartoma shows a large amount of fat (A) interspersed within glandular tissue (B). A very thin capsule is present.

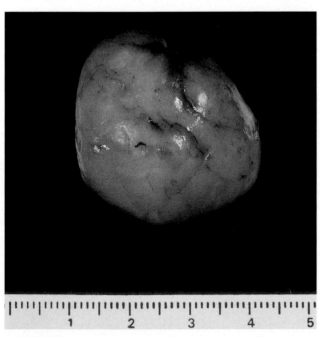

FIGURE 1.23

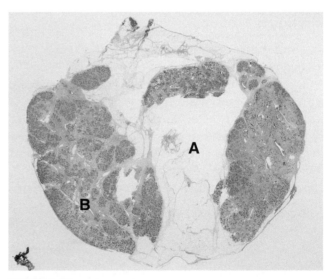

FIGURE 1.25

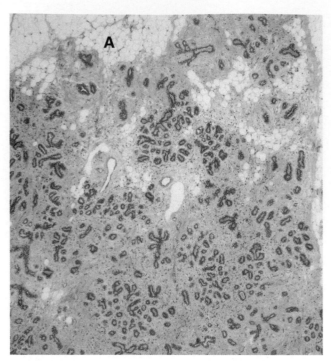

FIGURE 1.26

Figure 1.26

A histopathology section of the tumor shown in gross section in Figure 1.25 shows a large amount of fat (A) surrounding dense connective tissue, lobules, and ducts. The composition is similar to that of breast tissue, and for that reason, hamartomas have been described as "breast tissue within the breast."

TREATMENT

Hamartomas usually carry no serious potent. They may become larger, but not as large as fibroadenomas. Hamartomas are usually excised.

Phyllodes Tumor

In 1883, Johannes Mueller applied the name "cystosarcoma phyllodes" (from the Greek *sarkos* ["flesh"]) to a large breast tumor that had a fleshy appearance, with intratumoral cystic formations. The term "cystosarcoma" has been misleading and confusing because "sarcoma" implies a malignant tumor. Today, the name has been changed to phyllodes tumor [from the Greek *phyllos* ("leaves")] because of the "leaf" appearance of the tumor on microscopic examination.

CLINICAL PRESENTATION

Phyllodes tumors are relatively uncommon. They account for 0.3%–0.5% of all breast tumors in women. Phyllodes tumors rarely occur in men. When they do, they may arise from a gynecomastia.

The age incidence for phyllodes tumor is between 35 and 55 years.

When small, phyllodes tumors, like fibroadenomas, are asymptomatic. As a phyllodes tumor becomes larger, the patient may complain of soreness in the breast. When the tumor is superficially located, the contour of the breast may have a lobulated appearance.

Sometimes, however, the clinical presentation can be dramatic. The patient may state that she has had a tumor in her breast for a long time, and that suddenly the tumor has rapidly increased in size. As that change occurs, the patient begins to feel that her brassiere has become tight and that the breast has become painful.

The size change can be insidious or very rapid, taking only a few months. As the tumor becomes larger, mastodynia ensues. The patient starts to have soreness, heaviness, and finally pain that is unrelated to the menstrual cycle. Nipple discharge is not a common symptom.

When a phyllodes tumor grows to a large size, the overlying skin becomes thinner and shiny. The tumor may undergo central necrosis, resulting in cyst formation. (That is the reason phyllodes tumors were previously called "*cysto*sarcomas.")

A cyst that develops within a phyllodes tumor is unlike a simple cyst of the breast. Whereas the surface of a simple cyst is smooth, cystic formation within a phyllodes tumor is lobulated, and some areas "ballot" and "feel cystic." The tumor has a solid consistency on palpation, but if the breast is moved using bimanual palpation, the examiner perceives an "oscillatory" noise resulting from the movement of the fluid within the tumor. The fluid is usually thick and darkish brown-green in color, quite different from the thinner and lighter-colored fluid seen in the simple cysts of fibrocystic disease.

Phyllodes tumors are usually unilateral. Only a few cases of synchronous bilateral disease have been described.

PHYSICAL EXAMINATION

When a clinical history or follow-up examination indicates that a tumor has become larger in a relatively short period (months), a diagnosis of phyllodes tumor should be suspected.

Figure 1.27

Figure 1.27 shows a 21-year-old patient who noted a tumor on her right breast during self-examination. The increase in size occurred within a two-month period. The patient had no other symptoms such as pain or nipple discharge.

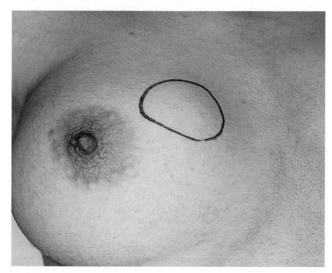

FIGURE 1.27

On physical examination, the tumor was located in the upper inner quadrant of the right breast. The tumor measured approximately 3 cm and was not tender. A loss of breast contour was noted during the inspection as the patient raised her arms. On palpation, the surface of the tumor was smooth and lobulated.

Because of the rapid growth, a diagnosis of phyllodes tumor was suspected.

Figure 1.28
Phyllodes tumors lack a true capsule. Although the tumor's margin may appear intact on the gross specimen, microscopic infiltrations to the adjacent

breast tissue generally occur. Figure 1.28 shows the gross specimen of the phyllodes tumor from the patient shown in Figure 1.27. The tumor was lobulated. The lobulations could be felt during the physical examination.

Figures 1.29 and 1.30
Surgeons should become familiar with the gross appearance of a phyllodes tumor so that the tumor can be recognized during a surgical procedure.

Two specimens – a fibroadenoma (Figure 1.29) and a phyllodes tumor (Figure 1.30) – are bisected for didactic purposes. The fibroadenoma has a smooth cut surface and a firm consistency. A definite capsule can be appreciated (arrow). The gross specimen of a phyllodes tumor lacks a capsule, and the surface of the tumor has a lobulated, fleshy appearance.

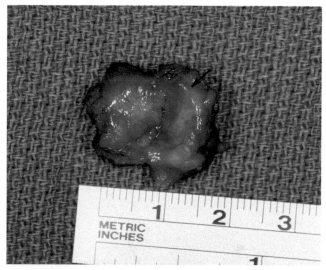

FIGURE 1.29

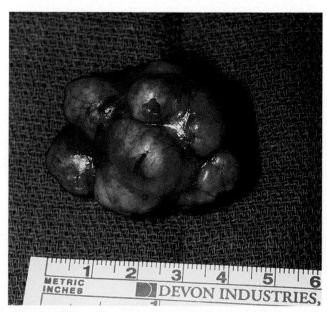

FIGURE 1.28

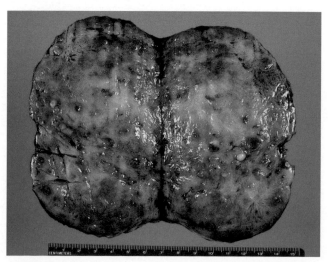

FIGURE 1.30

A frozen section should always be done if a clinical diagnosis of phyllodes tumor is suspected. If the frozen section diagnosis concurs with the clinical diagnosis, then a wider excision of normal breast tissue should be done at that moment. Failure to do so will result in local recurrence.

If a diagnosis of phyllodes tumor cannot be made from the frozen section, but is then confirmed from the permanent sections, the patient must be informed. Re-excision should be recommended.

Figure 1.31

Phyllodes tumors are usually single. Bilateral synchronous or metachronous phyllodes tumors are rare; however, the author has documented a few such cases. Figure 1.31 shows one patient with such a presentation.

The 52-year-old patient had noted progressive enlargement of both breasts. There was no history of mastodynia, but the patient stated that her brassiere had become tight and that, by the time she noticed the tumors, she was having some discomfort bilaterally (described as soreness and heaviness).

The tumors measured approximately 10 cm in diameter. A core biopsy confirmed the clinical diagnosis of benign phyllodes tumor.

The patient was treated with wide local excisions followed by bilateral augmentation mammoplasty. (The surgical technique is described in chapter 11, "Excision of Multiple and Large Benign Breast Tumors)."

Figure 1.32

Clinically, as a phyllodes tumor grows, loss of breast contour becomes more apparent, and lobulation becomes more pronounced. This physical find-

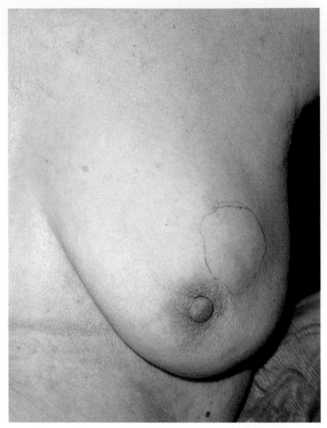

FIGURE 1.32

ing can be emphasized by conducting the inspection with the patient pressing hands to hips.

Figure 1.33

When a phyllodes tumor is located deep in the breast, the lobulated surface may not be visible. In Figure 1.33 marked asymmetry (enlarged left breast)

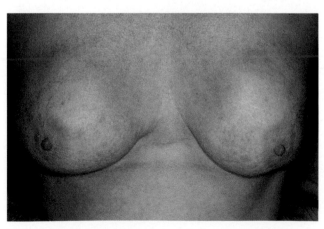

FIGURE 1.31

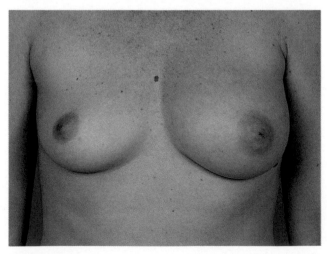

FIGURE 1.33

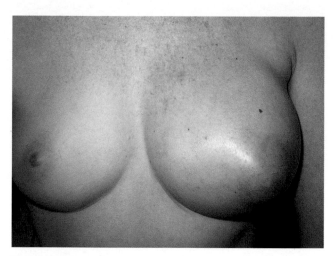

FIGURE 1.34

is seen. A phyllodes tumor was suspected because of a history of rapid growth.

Figure 1.34

A phyllodes tumor may arise from a preexisting fibroadenoma. The 48-year-old patient in Figure 1.34 gave a history of having had a tumor on her left breast for several years. The patient stated that she noted her left breast becoming larger and her brassiere tight. She also complained of mastodynia. Three months had lapsed between the start of the symptoms and the time of the consultation.

On physical examination, marked asymmetry was evident. The left breast was very large (estimated to be three times the size of the right breast). On palpation, a well-defined tumor was found to occupy the central portion of the left breast. The tumor measured approximately 12 cm in diameter. Its surface was smooth and not lobulated. The consistency was firm. A core biopsy confirmed the diagnosis of benign phyllodes tumor.

To prevent a large frontal scar, the tumor was excised via the Gaillard–Thomas incision as explained in "Excision of Multiple and Large Benign Tumors" in chapter 11, "Surgical Treatment of Benign Breast Lesions."

IMAGING

Radiographically, distinguishing between malignant and benign phyllodes tumors and giant fibroadenomas is often difficult. On mammography examination, a phyllodes tumor images with a homogenous shadow. Fibroadenomas image with a smoother contour; phyllodes tumors are slightly lobulated.

On ultrasound examination, an uncomplicated phyllodes tumor may image in exactly the same way as a fibroadenoma. In other cases, the internal architecture may show cystic spaces and nonhomogenous echo texture. Ultrasonography can be used to confirm the development of intratumoral cysts.

Tissue sampling is required for a definitive diagnosis. A core biopsy is more helpful than a fine-needle aspiration biopsy in determining the nature of the lesion. The sampling can also be done by stereotactic mammotome or ultrasound-guided biopsy.

CLINICAL-PATHOLOGY CORRELATION

This section discusses only the clinical progression of unattended phyllodes tumor, whether benign or malignant. Histopathology is discussed in chapter 9, "Role of the Pathologist."

Figure 1.35

If not properly excised benign phyllodes tumor can recur. The 58-year-old patient in Figure 1.35 was seen in consultation three years after having had surgery on her left breast. She had been told that the tumor was "benign." She was asymptomatic, but consulted because she noted that her left breast had become progressively larger.

The original pathology slides were reviewed, and the diagnosis of benign phyllodes tumor was confirmed.

On physical examination, a scar in the upper outer quadrant from the prior breast surgery was noted. A loss of the normal breast contour had occurred because a large lobulated mass occupied the entire upper outer quadrant and extending to the upper inner and lateral

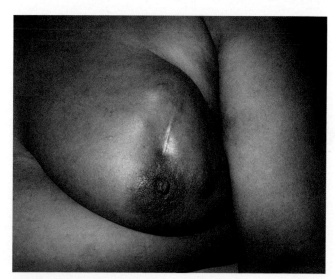

FIGURE 1.35

quadrants of the left breast. The skin was shiny, but no skin dimpling or nipple retraction was seen. On palpation, the lobulation was uniformly smooth. The consistency was firm but "spongy."

A core breast biopsy confirmed the clinical suspicion of recurrent benign phyllodes tumor.

Although the tumor was benign, the wide excision required for a tumor of this size in a relatively normal-sized breast would have left an undesirable deformity. The patient was treated with a total mastectomy.

Figure 1.36

In Figure 1.36, clinical differential diagnosis had to distinguish a carcinoma from a large, lobulated phyllodes tumor.

The patient had a large malignant tumor on the left breast. The mass was hard in consistency and fixed to the subcutaneous tissue and the skin. Fixation as a physical sign is important for the differential diagnosis between a large lobulated carcinoma and a large lobulated phyllodes tumor. Phyllodes tumors may extend to the adjacent tissue, but they displace those tissues rather than infiltrate them.

Differentiating between benign and malignant phyllodes tumors is difficult not only clinically but also histopathologically. See chapter 9, "Role of the Pathologist" for the histopathology description.

Figure 1.37

Figure 1.37 shows the condition of a 65-year-old woman who consulted because of the "foul odor" emanating from her left breast. She could not tell when the breast started to have this clinical presentation.

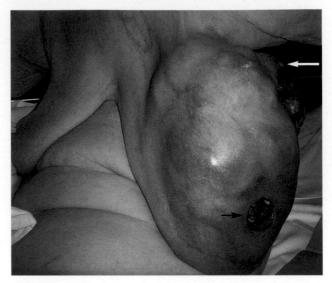

FIGURE 1.37

The left breast was approximately five times the size of the right. The skin surface was shiny and red. A fungating mass occupied the upper quadrant, and the nipple was completely eroded (arrow). The surface of the breast was lobulated. On palpation the tumor was firm in consistency with some areas of fluctuation. When the breast was moved bimanually, an "oscillatory" noise could be elicited. This auditory effect had a resonance similar to that produced when a coconut is moved side to side.

The patient was treated with a total mastectomy (the so-called cleansing mastectomy) (see "Surgical Treatment of Malignant Breast Lesions," Figure 12.65). The pathology diagnosis was consistent with benign phyllodes tumor.

The clinical presentation of this patient well illustrates the progression that can occur with untreated phyllodes tumor. As the tumor increases in size, the skin thins. Its color may change to reddish with a cyanotic hue. The tumor does not adhere to the skin. (If a surgical probe is placed between the tumor and the subcutaneous tissue, the two tissue planes can be separated.)

When a phyllodes tumor becomes larger, tumor necrosis may occur. The necrosis may result either from intratumoral bleeding or from compression of the blood supply. (The compression is caused by the size of the tumor and not by direct extension of the tumor into the skin, as occurs in carcinoma.) When the tumor is superficial, the compression may cause the skin to necrotize and ulcerate (small and large arrows). In deeper tumors, the necrotized tissue eventually liquefies, resulting in a cystic formation. At

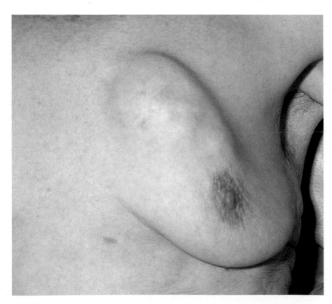

FIGURE 1.36

that stage, moving the breast during a physical examination gives an oscillatory noise, and palpation gives a "spongy" consistency.

The clinical differential diagnosis that should be entertained is with an inflammatory carcinoma. In inflammatory carcinoma, the skin becomes edematous and thickened, and the skin pores distend, giving the skin the appearance of an orange rind *(peau d'orange)*. (See chapter 2, "Malignant Tumors.")

Figure 1.38

Figure 1.38 demonstrates the clinical presentation of a malignant phyllodes tumor. This 55-year-old patient gave a history of having had surgery on her left breast several years before the current clinical presentation. The patient stated that her left breast had become progressively larger and that she was having mastodynia. There was no nipple discharge.

On clinical examination, marked asymmetry was noted. The left breast was between three and four times the size of the right. A scar from a previous biopsy was evident in the upper quadrant of the left breast. The skin was shiny and thin. It had a reddish color with a cyanotic hue. There were prominent superficial veins, but no skin dimpling or nipple retraction.

The surface of the tumor was lobulated, smooth, and hard. No fixation to the subcutaneous tissue or to the pectoralis muscle was noted. A core biopsy revealed this tumor to be a malignant phyllodes tumor.

The records of the previous surgery on the left breast were not available. It could therefore never be established whether the original tumor had been benign or malignant.

DIFFERENTIAL DIAGNOSIS OF LARGE BREAST LESIONS

Large, uncomplicated phyllodes tumors should be differentiated from giant fibroadenomas, giant lipomas, large malignant tumors, and sarcomas.

Phyllodes tumors occur in middle-aged patients. They may grow rapidly to a large size in a short time. Because they do not infiltrate to the surrounding breast tissue, they are not fixed.

Giant fibroadenomas occur in younger patients (see Figure 1.19 earlier in this chapter.) They grow slowly and are mobile. Phyllodes tumors and giant fibroadenomas are both firm in consistency, but the surface of a phyllodes tumor is lobulated, whereas the surface of a giant fibroadenoma is smooth.

Giant lipomas occur mostly in older patients. They grow insidiously and are soft on palpation.

Figures 1.39 and 1.40

The 66-year-old patient in Figure 1.39 had a large tumor on her right breast. The breast became progressively larger over the course of several years. The patient had no symptoms.

On inspection, asymmetry of the breast was seen to be due to a large tumor located in both upper quadrants of the right breast. The tumor became more prominent when the patient pressed both hands against her hips. (With the latter maneuver, the chest muscles contract, and because of its origin it protrudes through the muscle fibers.) The surface of the tumor was smooth and well circumscribed. On palpation, the consistency was soft.

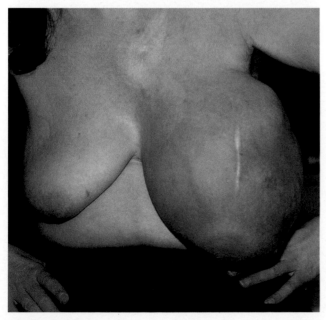

FIGURE 1.38

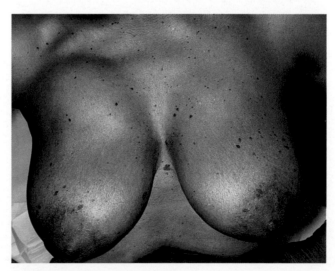

FIGURE 1.39

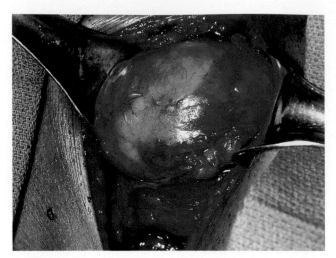

FIGURE 1.40

At surgery, the lipoma was found to originate from the fat between the pectoralis minor and major muscles. The pectoralis muscle fibers were split to gain access to the lipoma (Figure 1.40). (Lipomas in the breast area develop from the fat between the pectoralis major and pectoralis minor muscles, and *not* from the subcutaneous tissue adjacent to the breast parenchyma.)

Figure 1.41
Primary malignant fibrohistiocytomas of the breast are rare. When the patient in Figure 1.41 was seen in 1985, only 143 cases had been reported in the world literature. The clinical presentation and physical findings were quite similar to those of a phyllodes tumor.

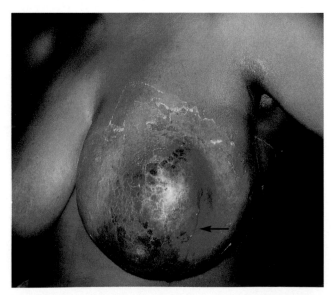

FIGURE 1.41

The 45-year-old patient noted discoloration on the skin of her left breast three years before discovering a lump. She had no mastodynia or nipple discharge at that time. Two weeks before the consultation, she developed a sudden enlargement of the left breast and left mastodynia. This latter symptom suddenly subsided with a breakage of the skin and spontaneous drainage of a large amount of serosanguineous fluid (Figure 1.41, arrow). At the time of the consultation, serous-colored fluid was still draining. The breast was practically occupied by a hard, lobulated tumor measuring 10 cm in its greatest diameter. Although the tumor was hard in consistency, an area of fluctuation was noted at its center. Palpation of that area resulted in a gush of serosanguineous fluid. A large lymph node was palpable on the left axilla.

Figure 1.42
Figure 1.42 shows the mammogram for the patient in Figure 1.41. Pockets of air (arrows) are present in the tumor. The air most likely came from exposure of the tumor to the outside via the fistula. The diagnosis of malignant fibrous histiocytoma was made on incisional biopsy. The patient was treated

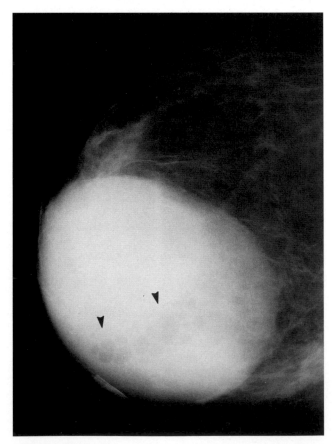

FIGURE 1.42

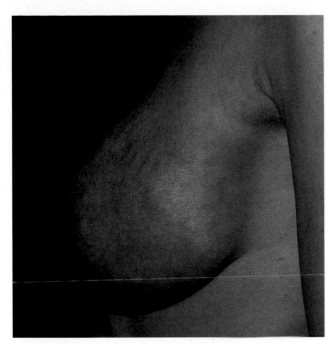

FIGURE 1.43

with a total mastectomy with low axillary node dissection. No axillary metastasis was found.

Figure 1.43

Primary lymphoma of the breast is rare. It constitutes 0.12%–0.53% of all breast malignancies and 10%–20.6% of sarcomas of the breast.

The 48-year-old patient in Figure 1.43 presented with a one-month history of a rapidly enlarging left breast. Marked venous dilatation and distension of the skin of the left breast were noted. The tumor was located in the upper outer quadrant of the left breast. It measured approximately 6 cm, and was hard, irregular, and fixed to the surrounding breast tissue. No *peau d'orange*, dimpling of the skin, nipple retraction, or discharge was seen.

Preoperative needle aspiration cytology revealed anaplastic cell nuclei consistent with a neoplastic process. The mammogram was nonspecific. Frozen-section diagnosis was consistent with a medullary carcinoma. The diagnosis of primary lymphoma of the breast was confirmed with permanent paraffin sections. Inmunoperoxidase stain confirmed the lymphoreticular origin of the lesion.

TREATMENT

Treatment of phyllodes tumors depends on the patient's age, the tumor size, and whether the tumor is benign or malignant. Small benign phyllodes tumors are treated with local excision. A wide rim of normal breast tissue is taken to ensure complete tumor removal and to prevent a local recurrence. Large, complicated, benign phyllodes tumors should be treated with a total mastectomy, as should multiple local recurrences that have already resulted in a deformed breast.

Malignant phyllodes tumors metastasize through the bloodstream. A complete axillary node dissection is therefore unnecessary. These tumors are treated with a total mastectomy and low axillary dissection to ensure complete removal of the breast, including the tail of Spence (axillary breast extension).

The various surgical techniques for excision of phyllodes tumors are described in chapter 11, "Surgical Treatment of Benign Breast Lesions."

FIBROCYSTIC CHANGES

The histologic breast findings commonly called "fibrocystic disease" have been a clinical problem for many years. That problem is reflected in the various names that the clinical entity has received in the past: for example, chronic cystic mastitis, benign cystic disease, Schimmelbusch disease, maladies kystiques des mammelles, and Reclus disease, among others. Because this entity is now considered to be a physiologic rather than a pathologic condition, the name "fibrocystic changes" was assigned at the Consensus Conference of the College of American Pathologists in 1985.

The cytoarchitecture of the mammary gland is known to follow a dynamic pattern that changes during the phases of the menstrual cycle. These histologic changes occur throughout a woman's reproductive life, starting at puberty and ceasing at menopause.

At puberty, the physiologic mechanism of the changes is initiated by the hypothalamus, which stimulates the secretion of follicle stimulating hormone (FSH) and luteinizing hormone (LH) from the anterior pituitary gland. The increase of FSH/LH activates the secretion of estrogen from the primordial ovarian follicles. The estrogen is responsible for initial development of the breast, including the growth of the connective tissue and the increase in vascularity that supports the newly formed ducts. Progesterone is responsible for the development of the lobules that sprout from the terminal ductal buds.

The fluctuation in the various elements of the breast parenchyma that occurs throughout the menstrual cycle varies with the age of the woman. The lobular units are at their most numerous in the third

decade of life. It is at that age and in a woman's mid to late forties that advanced clinical fibrocystic changes such as pronounced nodularity, lumpiness, and macrocysts occur.

At menopause, the breast becomes pendulous, the lobules atrophy and become smaller, and the connective tissue is almost replaced by fat. The atrophic lobular units – which maintain a firm consistency – contrast markedly with the soft consistency of the surrounding fat. That contrast explains the "increased nodularity" clinical finding in menopausal patients.

CLINICAL PRESENTATION

The symptoms of fibrocystic changes are pain, nodularity, a dominant mass, cysts, and (occasionally) nipple discharge. Breast pain (mastodynia) and a clinical finding of nodularity or tissue thickening are the characteristic signs of fibrocystic changes.

The patient's description of the pain can range from "discomfort" to "excruciating." The severity of the symptom is related to the degree of swelling and to the patient's pain threshold, rather than to the histologic findings.

Mammary blood flow is well known to increase as an estrogen effect that is maximal at the end of each menstrual cycle, increasing breast volume and the associated mastodynia. The pain commences by the second week of each cycle. It becomes maximal three to seven days before the menses begin and progressively decreases in severity during the two to three days following the menses.

The cause of the pain should be well explained to the patient. Otherwise, if she is told that she has a "disease," unnecessary anxiety may magnify the symptoms.

Although breast pain certainly carries the highest degree of suspicion of fibrocystic changes, other conditions must also be considered. These include

- intercostal neuralgia,
- stretching of the Cooper's ligaments (associated with large, pendulous breasts),
- Tietze's syndrome (costochondralgia), and
- trauma (also see chapter 3, "Pain").

The various histologic patterns that the breast exhibits during the physiologic changes have common features:

- proliferation of the cell or fibrous components, leading to cystic changes

- changes associated with ductal or lobular hyperplasia
- alterations of the stroma, particularly fibrosis

Based on the histologic patterns (singly or in combination), the most common fibrocystic changes are

- microcyst and macrocyst ("blue dome cyst"),
- adenosis (florid, blunt, and sclerosing adenosis),
- fibrosis,
- duct ectasia, and
- intraductal and lobular hyperplasia.

These histomorphologic changes should not be considered pathologic, but rather local findings. They may be shown at biopsy (in patients operated on either because of the severity of their symptoms or because of clinical findings) or in breast tissue removed in the process of a lumpectomy or mastectomy.

PHYSICAL EXAMINATION

This subsection discusses microcysts, adenosis, fibrosis, duct ectasia, and hyperplasias. Because macrocysts require a different approach to treatment, they are discussed in their own section (see "Macrocysts" later in this chapter).

PATHOGENESIS
Microcyst

Microcysts are microscopic – less than 1 mm in size – and are therefore nonpalpable. They are found mainly in breast tissue excised in the process of a lumpectomy or mastectomy. Microcystic changes are the most common finding in the breast – to the point that they are considered to be within the spectrum of normality.

Figure 1.44

Microcysts develop at the level of the terminal duct lobular component (TDLC) of the breast (see chapter 2, "Malignant Tumors," Figure 2.13). They are the result of an obstruction of the terminal duct as it enters the acinus. The obstruction is a combination of cell and fibrous-tissue proliferation and of secretion from active acinar epithelial tissue.

Owing to the hormonal imbalance just before and during the onset of menopause, the acinar epithelium desquamates and liquefies, resulting in accumulation of secretions within the acinus. As the secretion accumulates, the acinus distends, producing a thinning of its epithelial lining. Some of the accumulated secretions may leak through the now thinner acinar wall,

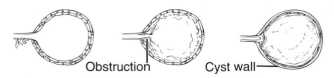

FIGURE 1.44

producing chronic inflammation and fibrosis. The inflammatory process thickens the stroma around the cyst, resulting in formation of a "wall." The obstruction progresses until it becomes complete.

Figure 1.45

Figure 1.45 shows a residual lobular acinus to the left of a developing microcyst. The secretions of the apocrine epithelium and desquamation of some epithelial cells of the acini produce an obstruction at the junction of the terminal tubule and the acini (arrow). That process initiates dilation of the acini, leading to formation of a microcyst (A). When apocrine secretion continues, the microcyst increases in size to form a macrocyst (see Figure 1.49).

Adenosis

Adenosis results from proliferation of the epithelium and myoepithelium of the lobules and terminal ductule, or changes in the amount of fibrous tissue, or both. The coalescent lobules may form a mass – thus the name "adenosis tumor," which has also been given to this type of fibrocystic change. (See Figures 9.15 through 9.17 in chapter 9, "Role of the Pathologist.")

Blunt adenosis is more commonly present in younger patients (women in their thirties or early forties). Sclerosing adenosis (see Figures 9.18 and 9.19 in chapter 9, "Role of the Pathologist") occurs in patients in their fourth and fifth decades.

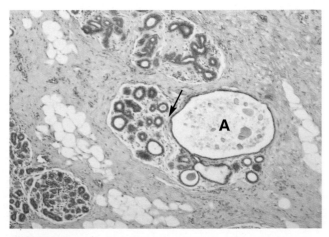

FIGURE 1.45

Clinically, as for all histologic forms of fibrocystic change, pain is present. The pain is cyclical. On examination, florid adenosis and blunt adenosis manifest with a firm nodularity. Multiple nodules are usually found. They may be confined to one area of one breast ("local adenosis") or they may be dispersed within one quadrant ("multifocal adenosis") or among several quadrants in both breasts ("multicentric adenosis").

On palpation, the examiner has a sense of touching small pebbles or a bunch of chickpeas lying on a flat surface. The nodules are slightly tender to palpation (see chapter 6, "The Role of The Clinician").

When an area of adenosis is accompanied by stroma proliferation or reactive fibrosis, the condition is called sclerosing adenosis. The nodules then become more prominent, more defined, and firmer or harder in consistency.

Sclerosing adenosis may calcify. Typically, the calcifications associated with sclerosing adenosis are large and scattered throughout the breast. The configuration differs from the calcification seen in ductal carcinoma in situ, in which the calcifications are clustered and irregular. (See chapter 8, "Role of the Radiologist.")

Duct Ectasia

Duct ectasia occurs mostly in premenopausal patients. It is the result of glandular involution and secretory retention in the ducts. As a result, the major ducts enlarge. With time, the secretions may penetrate the duct wall, resulting in an associated periductal inflammatory reaction.

When secretions accumulate, the patient starts to complain of fullness and a burning sensation in the nipple area. The burning sensation may lead a patient to squeeze her nipples, finding a thick discharge (Figure 1.46). This discharge is non-spontaneous, intermittent, and of diverse color (ranging from yellow initially to orange when it becomes chronic).

In the initial stage of duct ectasia, the areola skin may be red and edematous. In the chronic stage, the involved duct becomes thicker and feels tubular, tortuous, and "wormlike." (Bloodgood coined the name "varicocele of the breast" for this condition. See Figure 1.47) Chronically inflamed retroareolar ducts may cause nipple retraction (Figure 1.48).

Figure 1.46

Figure 1.46 demonstrates nipple discharge in a patient with chronic duct ectasia. The discharge is always provoked (non-spontaneous). Its consistency

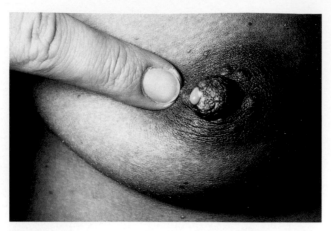

FIGURE 1.46

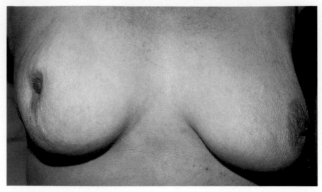

FIGURE 1.48

is thick, and its color can vary among yellow, white, and brown – singly or in combination.

Figure 1.47

Figure 1.47 shows a dilated duct (arrow) in a case of duct ectasia. The affected ducts are usually the terminal major ducts located under the areola. When dilation is accompanied by periductal inflammation, the palpatory sensation resembles that of a varicocele or thrombosed vein.

Figure 1.48

Figure 1.48 shows nipple retraction resulting from chronic duct ectasia. This retraction differs from the retraction caused by a malignant process. With a malignancy, the retracted nipple may be accompanied by skin dimpling and a hard retroareolar mass. The nipple can not be everted. When the retraction is caused by chronic duct ectasia the nipple can partially be everted.

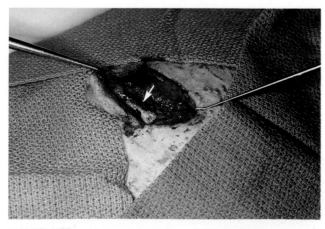

FIGURE 1.47

TREATMENT

Because fibrocystic changes of the breast are physiologic rather than pathologic, they generally require no surgical treatment (but see "Macrocysts" later in this chapter for an exception). After a careful physical examination, imaging, and fine-needle aspiration biopsy, patients with fibrocystic changes may be treated medically.

Medical treatment options range from those that merely relieve symptoms (such as diuretics) to those that may counteract the physiologic effects of estrogen production (such as progestogens [progesterone and progesterone derivatives], progestin [19-nortestosterone derivatives], androgens [danazol], antiestrogen [tamoxifen], antiprolactin [bromocriptine], abstinence from or lower intake of methylxanthines [tea, coffee, chocolate], and vitamins E and B).

Diuretics

Diuretics treat only the symptoms. They are used toward the end of the menstrual cycle, when breast volume increases owing to water retention.

Oral Contraceptives

The effectiveness of oral contraceptives in alleviating breast pain is based on their action in reducing ovarian estradiol production, which is modulated in breast tissue by its progesterone component.

Danazol (17-alpha-norethisterone)

Danazol is an androgen derivative. Its action in relieving symptoms of fibrocystic changes is related to its inhibitory effect: it competitively inhibits the binding of sex steroids to receptors. Because of its side effects, danazol is infrequently used. Among its listed side effects are vaginal spotting, nausea, headache, muscle cramps, depression, and virilization. Danazol is contraindicated in patients with abnormal hepatic, renal, or cardiac function.

Tamoxifen

Tamoxifen, an estrogen antagonist, has been reported to be useful in treating patients with fibrocystic change. Because tamoxifen induces symptoms of menopause, use of this medication is reserved for symptomatic perimenopausal patients.

Bromocriptine

The use of bromocriptine (Parlodel) in the treatment of fibrocystic change assumes a role for prolactin in the development of the condition. The author has had clinical experience of patients with fibrocystic symptoms and signs who were treated with Parlodel for infertility with no benefit to the breast.

Methylxanthines

Choosing to reduce consumption of methylxanthines (contained in caffeine) is based on studies by Minton (1988, 1989). Methylxanthines are thought to inhibit normal-cycle adenosine monophosphate phosphodiesterase and guanosine monophosphate phosphodiesterase action with concomitant increase in cyclic adenosine monophosphate and cyclic guanosine monophosphate. Increased intracellular monophosphate is believed to stimulate protein kinase, resulting in proliferation of cystic breast tissue.

Vitamins

The use of certain vitamins – specifically vitamins E and B – while restricting intake of methylxanthines has been suggested as potentially beneficial in reducing the symptoms of fibrocystic change. Minton reported a 65% reduction in symptoms in a small series of patients treated with such a regime.

MACROCYSTS

Macrocysts are the most common benign breast mass in women. Clinically symptomatic cysts occur in approximately 7% of all women. The incidental finding of cysts in patients who undergo surgery for other causes is about 25%.

CLINICAL PRESENTATION

Like fibroadenomas, macrocysts are three-dimensional entities. They differ from fibroadenomas only in their content: while fibroadenomas are solid, cysts contain fluid.

Figure 1.49
Large cysts are thin-walled and bluish in color – hence the alternative name "blue dome cyst".

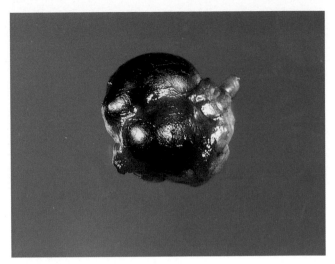

FIGURE 1.49

Cysts are more common in middle-aged women (aged 40–50 years). The incidence decreases after menopause, unless the patient is on hormone replacement therapy – in which case, the incidence may continue as long as exogenous hormones are being administered.

In general, cysts are asymptomatic. Sometimes, however, a sudden pain in the breast draws the patient's attention to a mass. The pain is associated with the sudden accumulation of fluid.

The patient may describe the pain as "sharp," "dull," "burning sensation," or "fullness." The pain and sensation of fullness are related to the rapid accumulation of fluid. The burning sensation is attributed to a chemical irritation resulting from some of the cyst content leaking into the surrounding breast tissue.

The combination of sudden pain and discovery of a lump frightens many women. Knowing this clinical presentation, the physician should be able to relieve the patient's anxiety at the beginning of the consultation.

PHYSICAL EXAMINATION

Like fibroadenomas, macrocysts are well delineated and have a smooth surface. Also like fibroadenomas, cysts can be solitary or multiple, and present in only one breast or bilaterally. Other physical characteristics of the cyst vary depending on the size of the cyst, the amount of fluid that it contains, and the degree of reaction that it causes in the surrounding breast tissue.

Figures 1.50 and 1.51
In general, the consistency of a cyst can be compared to a balloon filled with water (Figure 1.50) or

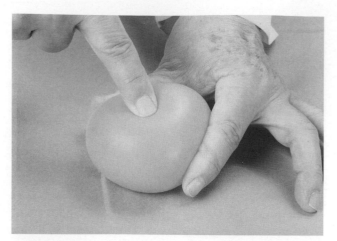

FIGURE 1.50

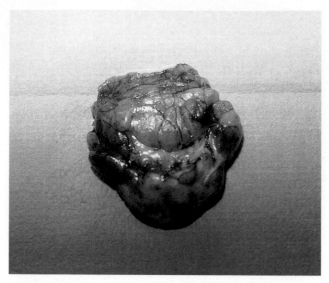

FIGURE 1.52

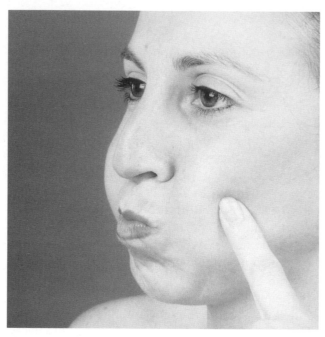

FIGURE 1.51

to a blown-out cheek (Figure 1.51). But the consistency can vary from soft through firm to hard, depending on the amount of fluid within the cyst.

Figure 1.52
When the fluid content is under pressure (a hard cyst), the consistency of the cyst may resemble that of a fibroadenoma or a cancer. A cluster of small cysts of this kind may present a hard, irregular surface (Figure 1.52).

Figure 1.53
A clinical differential diagnosis between a cyst and a solid tumor takes into account the fact that the

examiner's finger can displace ("ballot") the fluid within a cyst. Also, when the examiner presses the surface of a cyst, the patient may complain of tenderness in that area. Fibroadenomas and carcinomas are not tender on palpation.

Figure 1.54
Figure 1.54 demonstrates that the wall of a cyst is part of the breast parenchyma and not an independent entity as with fibroadenomas. The false sensation of mobility that the examiner perceives during the physical examination occurs because the cyst "moves" with the breast tissue to which it is incorporated.

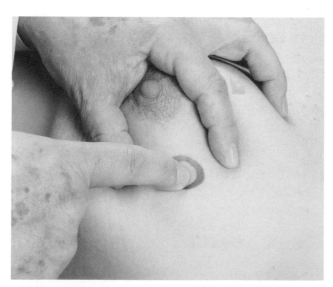

FIGURE 1.53

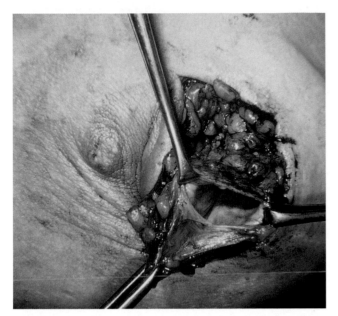

FIGURE 1.54

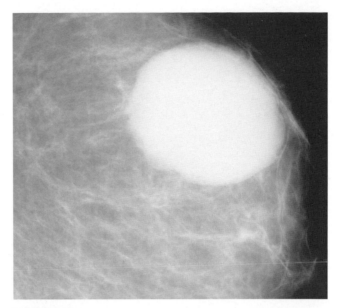

FIGURE 1.55

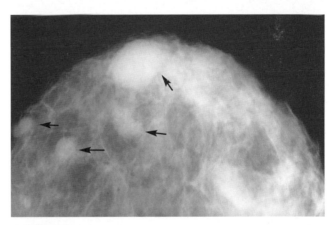

FIGURE 1.56

IMAGING

Mammography and ultrasonography of the breast are both quite accurate in differentiating a solid from a cystic tumor.

Figures 1.55 and 1.56

Like fibroadenomas, cysts image on a mammogram as round, ovoid, or lobulated masses. Depending on the amount of fluid in the cyst, density varies from low to high. If the fluid is abundant and under pressure, the cyst will have a density that may equal the density of a fibroadenoma. The difference between the image of a cyst and that of a fibroadenoma is that the latter demonstrates the so-called halo (see Figure 1.13 earlier in this chapter). The halo is the image of the "capsule" that surrounds the fibroadenoma.

This mediolateral oblique (MLO) mammographic projection in Figure 1.55 demonstrates a smoothly marginated mass (cyst) measuring 5 cm × 3 cm. The mammogram in Figure 1.56 images multiple cysts with varying densities because of the varying amount of fluid in each cyst (arrows).

Figures 1.57 and 1.58

On ultrasound examination, cysts usually image as anechoic lesions with a posterior enhancement. The cyst in Figure 1.57 is completely anechoic centrally (A). It has a thin, barely perceptible wall and demonstrates enhanced through-transmission posteriorly (B).

When the fluid in a cyst contains desquamated epithelial cells, the echo from the floating debris mimics a solid mass (Figure 1.58). A fine-needle aspiration FNA assists in differentiating such cysts from solid tumors.

TREATMENT

Macrocysts are usually treated by aspiration; surgery is rarely indicated. A cyst aspiration is an office or clinic procedure. A 22-gauge needle and a syringe of a size appropriate to the estimated cyst volume are used. Local anesthesia is unnecessary because the discomfort caused by a 22-gauge needle is minimal (about equal to the discomfort of a vein puncture). Stretching the skin overlying the cyst minimizes the discomfort caused by the needle puncture (see Figure 1.59 [arrows]).

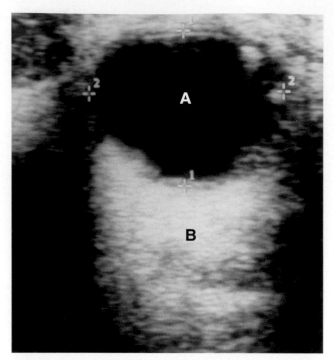

FIGURE 1.57

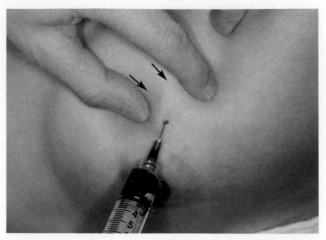

FIGURE 1.59

The cyst should be aspirated to dryness. With complete withdrawal of the fluid content, the cyst wall should collapse.

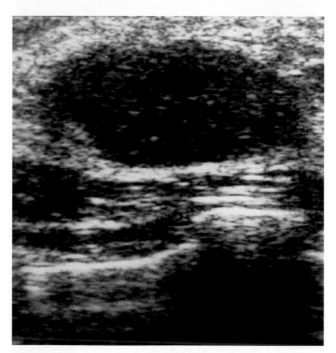

FIGURE 1.58

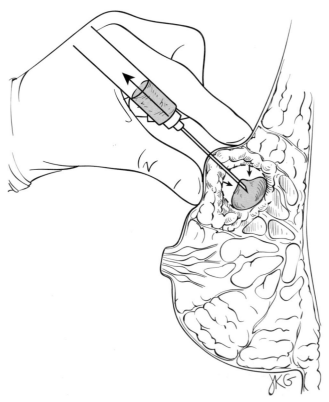

Figures 1.59 and 1.60

The skin is cleansed with alcohol, and the cyst is secured using the index finger and thumb of the non-dominant hand. As the fluid is being withdrawn, the physician should press down on the cyst with these two fingers.

FIGURE 1.60

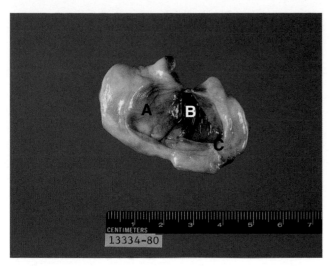

FIGURE 1.61

Figure 1.61

If the cyst is multilocular (A, B, C), passes in several directions may be required to aspirate every loculation.

Figure 1.62

When the cyst is large, a post-aspiration indentation can be felt at the site of the aspiration. That indentation represents the collapsed cyst wall. It is important to palpate the area thoroughly to discover any residual mass. If a residual mass is present, a fine-needle aspiration biopsy should be done on the mass.

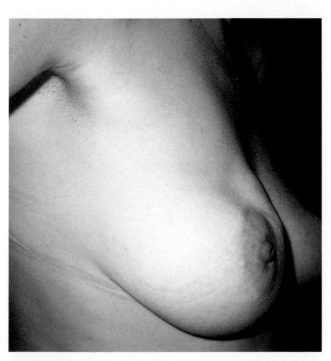

FIGURE 1.62

Figure 1.63

Figure 1.63 shows a specimen from a patient who had an intracystic tumor that became apparent post aspiration. (For illustrative purposes, the specimen was bisected.) The tumor is attached to the cyst wall by a wide pedicle (arrow). Because of the chronic nature of the cyst, its wall was thick.

The histopathology from the fine-needle aspiration biopsy was consistent with a benign intracystic papilloma. A differential diagnosis between benign and malignant intracystic papilloma can occasionally be made clinically on palpation by the consistency and contour of the mass. Benign intracystic papillomas are softer and well delineated; malignant intracystic papillomas are harder and poorly delineated.

Figures 1.64 and 1.65

The color of the aspirated fluid varies according to the age of the cyst or the underlying pathology, or both. The fluid of a recent cyst is yellowish (Figure 1.64), but with time changes to light brown, then dark green, and eventually black. The fluid may have a clear or turbid appearance (Figure 1.65). The turbidity depends on the amount of cell debris in the cyst. When the fluid is bloody, a papilloma or carcinoma should be suspected.

Figure 1.66

Milk cysts ("galactocele") should be suspected in a postpartum or lactating patient who develops pain and a mass on the breast (Figure 1.66). On physical examination, the mass is always tender. Blood-tinged

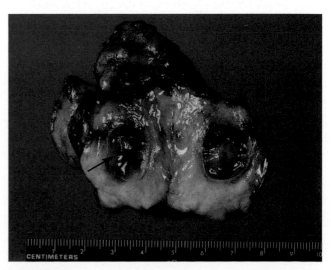

FIGURE 1.63

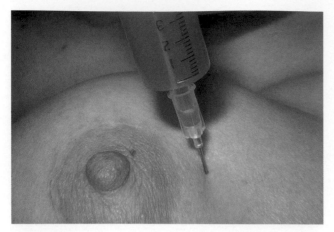

FIGURE 1.64

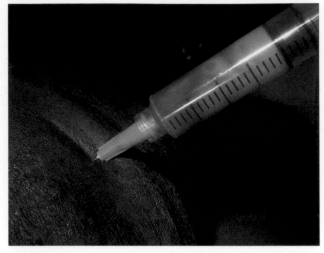

FIGURE 1.66

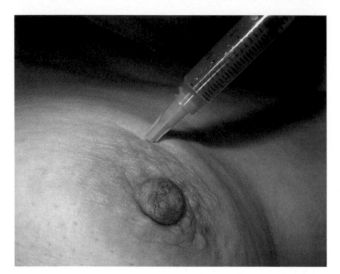

FIGURE 1.65

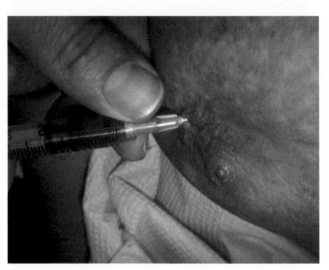

FIGURE 1.67

fluid is usually attributable to the breast engorgement that is common during pregnancy and lactation. It can also be the result of blood contamination from a punctured blood vessel.

Figure 1.67
Hemorrhage into a cyst may be idiopathic, secondary to an intracystic papilloma, or due to an intracystic papillary carcinoma. Hemorrhagic cysts should be excised regardless of whether the blood is fresh or old, and even when the cytology is negative.

Post-aspiration recurrence is not frequent, but it does occur. A cyst may recur immediately following aspiration or several days, weeks, or months later.

Recurrent cysts should be treated with re-aspiration. Excisional biopsy is recommended in cases of

- chronic reaccumulation
- hemorrhaged fluid
- positive cytology
- residual mass on completion of the aspiration
- abnormal post-aspiration mammogram

2

Malignant Tumors

Cancer is the second most common breast lesion after fibrocystic changes of the breast.

Breast cancer is asymptomatic. Malignant tumors are usually found on breast self-examination or during a routine physical examination. To be palpable, a tumor has to reach a size of 1 cm. In patients with large, pendulous breasts, detection of a tumor that size is difficult; the tumor may even be completely missed. But the increased use of screening mammography has resulted in more breast cancers being diagnosed in the subclinical stage – either as small, nonpalpable tumors or as microcalcifications.

BREAST CANCER OVERVIEW

In women, among all lesions of the breast, the incidence of cancerous lesions is 28%–30%. Although beast cancer has been diagnosed in patients in their late teens, the incidence at that age is low. Breast cancer reaches its highest incidence in patients between the ages of 45 and 50. The incidence declines somewhat in patients between the ages of 50 and 59, but then peaks again as the patient ages beyond 59 years.

CLINICAL PRESENTATION

Breast cancers are most commonly located in the upper outer quadrant of the breast – chiefly because that quadrant contains the greater volume of breast tissue. In order of decreasing frequency, the next most common locations are the upper inner, lower outer, and lower inner quadrants.

Cancer of the breast may appear as solitary, multiple, or bilateral tumors. The solitary type is more common. Bilateral cancers can be synchronous, or the second cancer may be diagnosed after the first (metachronous). Breast cancer occurs synchronously approximately 1% of the time and metachronously approximately 12%–15% of the time.

A distinction should be made between multicentric and multifocal breast cancer. In multifocal breast cancer, multiple primary cancer foci are found within one breast quadrant. In multicentric breast cancer, cancer foci develop in several quadrants of the breast.

PHYSICAL EXAMINATION

Characteristically, a breast cancer is a well-delineated tumor with irregular margins and a hard consistency. In the preclinical stage, breast cancer may manifest as a cluster of irregular heterogeneous microcalcifications; as a small, solitary, nonpalpable lesion; or as multiple lesions.

Certain physical findings may suggest the presence of a malignant mass. Those findings include changes in the skin (such as dimpling) or in the nipple (such as retraction or deviation).

On physical examination, some benign tumors present in a manner similar to that of a carcinoma. The most common of these are fat necrosis and granular cell tumors.

Fat necrosis results from trauma to the breast. It is a relatively uncommon breast lesion; but, being a hard and irregular tumor, it mimics a carcinoma. The consistency of the tumor comes from the collagenous scar that surrounds the lipid material released by lipocyte necrosis. A clinical history of trauma and the typical mammographic image of an "oil cyst" make the differential diagnosis (see chapter 8, "Role of the Radiologist," Figure 8.11).

Granular cell tumors are not specifically tumors of the breast; they can grow in any part of the body. Only 5% of granular cell tumors may be primary breast tumors. The physical findings are similar to those for breast carcinoma – that is, a hard and painless mass. When a granular cell tumor is superficially located or near the nipple, it may also, like a cancer, cause skin dimpling or nipple retraction, or both. Although granular cell tumors have been reported in adolescent and elderly women and in men, their occurrence is mainly in middle-aged women (40–50 years).

Figure 2.1
On physical examination, the solitary tumor in Figure 2.1 was well delineated, with irregular borders

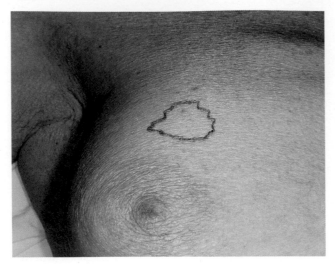

FIGURE 2.1

and a hard consistency. The clinical diagnosis is breast cancer.

Figures 2.2, 2.3, and 2.4
Several of the pleomorphic calcifications in Figure 2.2 show typical malignant branching. The final diagnosis was ductal carcinoma in situ.

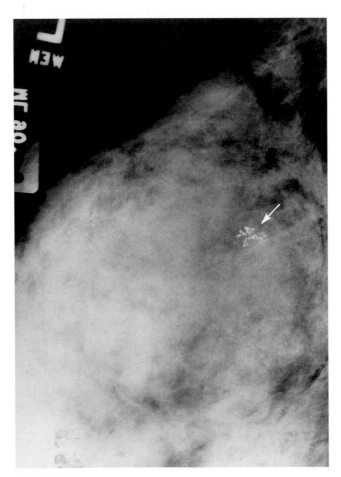

FIGURE 2.2

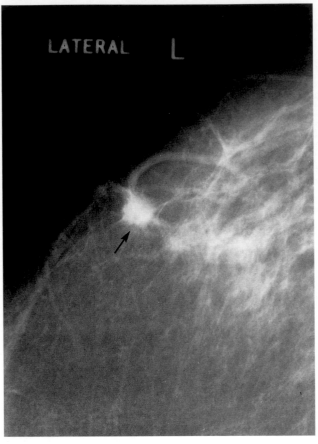

FIGURE 2.3

The lateral-view mammogram in Figure 2.3 images a 5-mm mass with a thin, spiculated margin. No associated microcalcifications are seen. The final diagnosis was infiltrating ductal carcinoma.

Figure 2.4 shows a multicentric carcinoma. This cranial-caudal (CC) projection mammogram demon-

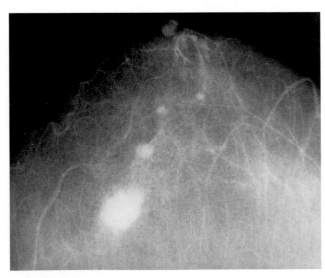

FIGURE 2.4

strates the presence of four lesions extending from the retroareolar region into the medial aspect of the breast. The largest lesion measures 8 mm in diameter, and the smallest, 3 mm in diameter. All have spiculated margins. The lesions are in different quadrants of the breast (multicentric).

Figures 2.5 and 2.6

Figure 2.5 shows the clinical presentation of a malignant tumor peripherally located in the left breast on the 3 o'clock radius. The skin dimpling became more apparent when the inspection was done with the patient's arms raised.

Figure 2.6 shows a locally advanced carcinoma located on the patient's left breast, just behind the areola at the nipple. Having the patient press hands against hips during the inspection produced this clinical sign.

Figures 2.7 and 2.8

Figure 2.7 is a gross specimen of a granular cell tumor of the breast (shown bisected). The tumor is well circumscribed. The irregular margins are due to infiltration of the tumor into the breast tissue. The infiltration was reflected in the physical examination: the tumor was irregular on palpation. The cut surface is grayish white in color. Notice the similarities between this benign tumor and an infiltrating ductal carcinoma (see Figure 2.10).

A mammogram on the cephalo-caudad (CC) view projection (Figure 2.8) and the medio lateral oblique (MLO) view (see Figure 8.25 in Chapter 8 "Role of the Radiologist") image the inferior and posterior location of the granular cell tumor shown in Figure 2.7. The tumor is partially obscured, indicating the need for good posterior depth in a mammography examination. The mass has serrated borders, which makes a mammographic differential diagnosis with infiltrating carcinoma difficult.

IMAGING

On mammography, cancers image with spiculated borders.

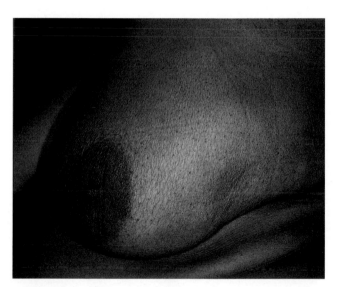

FIGURE 2.5

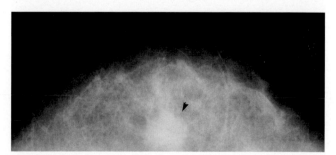

FIGURE 2.7

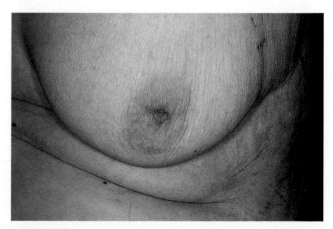

FIGURE 2.6

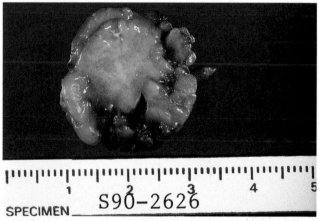

FIGURE 2.8

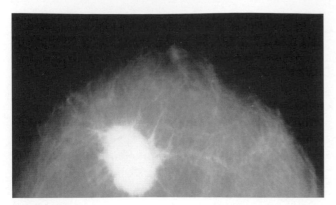

FIGURE 2.9

Figure 2.9

The mammogram in Figure 2.9 images the spiculated borders indicative of an infiltrating carcinoma (same patient shown in Figure 2.1).

PATHOLOGY

On gross examination the edges of an infiltrating carcinoma are "serrated" or "stellate" because as the malignancy grows and infiltrates, it radiates outward into the surrounding tissue.

Figure 2.10

In general, all breast specimens should be submitted intact to the pathologist for the evaluation of the margins. For teaching purposes, a gross specimen of an infiltrating carcinoma (Figure 2.10) tumor excised from the patient whose mammogram appears in Figure 2.9 was bisected to correlate the pathology with the physical examination and mammography findings. It shows "serrated" margins because the growing tumor radiates out into the surrounding breast parenchyma.

Figures 2.11 and 2.12

The histopathology findings for a granular cell tumor (Figures 2.11 and 2.12) show nests of sheets of spindle cells containing eosinophilic cytoplasmic granules. Granular cell tumors are not well marginated. To prevent a local recurrence, the excision should be widened into the normal-appearing breast tissue.

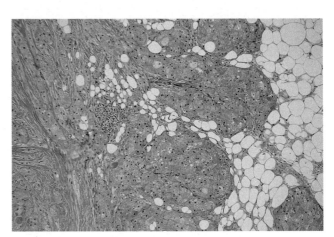

FIGURE 2.11

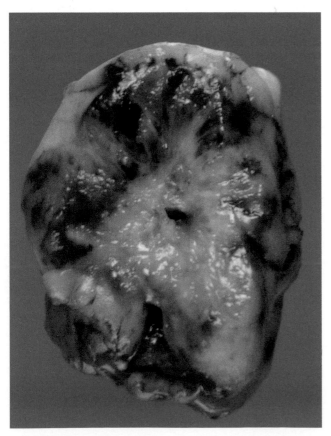

FIGURE 2.10

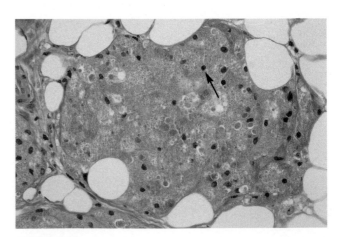

FIGURE 2.12

CLINICAL FEATURES OF IN SITU AND INVASIVE BREAST CANCER

Most breast cancers originate in the terminal duct lobular unit (TDLU). Because a malignancy can originate either from the ducts or from the lobules, breast cancer takes four major forms: ductal in situ, infiltrating ductal, lobular in situ (lobular neoplasia), and infiltrating lobular.

Other common invasive cancers are mucinous, medullary, papillary, and tubular. Those names derive from the pattern, morphology, and distribution of the associated cells. Two other unusual clinical presentations are Paget's disease of the nipple and inflammatory carcinoma.

Only the clinical aspects of these common types of breast cancer are discussed in this section; for the histopathology, see chapter 9, "Role of the Pathologist."

MICROANATOMY REVIEW

A brief review of the microanatomy of the breast may be helpful in understanding the clinical aspects of breast cancer.

The breast is composed of glandular tissue, fibrous tissue, and fat. All three components are distributed between fifteen and twenty lobes, which are separated one from the other by connective tissue.

Figure 2.13

Each lobe is an individual compound containing lobules (A). Each lobule contains acini (B), and each acinus drains into a small lactiferous duct. The junction of the acini and the small lactiferous duct is called DTLU (Terminal Duct Lobular Unit [C]). In a

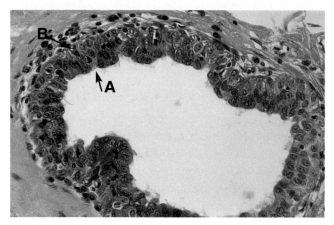

FIGURE 2.14

centrifugal fashion, the small lactiferous ducts progressively drain into larger ducts (D), each of which ends in a lactiferous sinus (E). Two or more lactiferous sinuses converge into a main duct which surfaces as an orifice at the skin (nipple).

Figure 2.14

Ducts and lobules both have two layers of cells: an epithelial inner layer (A) and a myoepithelial outer layer (B). The myoepithelial layer proliferates during pregnancy and lactation. Its function is to propel milk.

Breast cancer is designated "infiltrating" if the tumor cells have breached the myoepithelial layer and basement membrane.

In Situ Carcinomas

In situ carcinomas are those that have not infiltrated to the surrounding tissue.

DUCTAL CARCINOMA IN SITU

Before screening mammography, ductal carcinoma in situ (DCIS) was an uncommon breast lesion, accounting for only 2% of all lesions. With the increased use of screening mammography, DCIS now accounts for 15%–20% of all lesions. The lesion can be multicentric in 15%–38% of cases and bilateral in 10% of cases.

In the early stages, no physical signs are present. If the lesion remains undetected, a mass may eventually be palpable on clinical examination (Figure 2.15).

Although DCIS is usually diagnosed on mammography (imaged as a cluster of microcalcifications, see Figure 2.2), it may also be an incidental finding

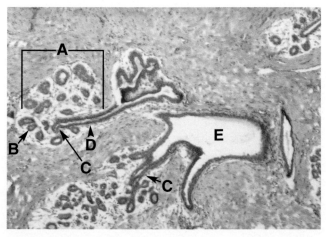

FIGURE 2.13

in breast tissue excised in the process of a lumpectomy for a benign lesion.

A higher incidence of DCIS is seen in patients between 45 years and 55 years of age.

Figures 2.15 and 2.16

Figure 2.15 shows a gross specimen of DCIS. This (palpable) lesion measured 0.8 cm. The arrow marks comedones protruding through the transected ducts. The comedones represent necrotic tissue resulting from an advanced in situ comedocarcinoma (Figure 2.16) (arrow).

LOBULAR CARCINOMA IN SITU

Lobular "carcinoma" is a misnomer. Haagensen (1986) gave lobular carcinoma in situ (LCIS) the name "lobular neoplasia" to avoid the clinical implications of the word "carcinoma." Lobular carcinoma in situ is now considered to be a marker. This histopathology finding marks a patient as being at high risk for developing invasive cancer of a ductal or lobular type.

The true incidence of LCIS is unknown, because it is usually an incidental finding in specimens

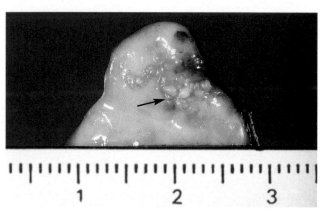

FIGURE 2.15

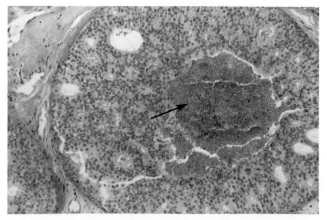

FIGURE 2.16

excised for other reasons. (Overall, lobular carcinomas constitute about 2.5% of all breast carcinomas.) Lobular carcinoma in situ is multicentric in about 40%–60% of cases and bilateral in 30%.

Unless an LCIS lesion is extensive, no specific clinical or mammographic features are evident.

The highest incidence of LCIS is seen in patients aged 40–50 years. The lesion is rarely seen after menopause – most likely because, at menopause, an involution of the breast lobules occurs, and LCIS may follow that pattern.

Invasive Carcinomas

The most common types of invasive breast cancer are infiltrating ductal and infiltrating lobular carcinoma. Other common invasive breast cancers are mucinous, medullary, papillary, and tubular carcinomas. These latter cancers are of ductal origin, but their names derive from the associated histologic features.

INFILTRATING DUCTAL CARCINOMA

Infiltrating ductal carcinoma is the most frequently seen invasive cancer. It accounts for 50%–70% of all invasive breast cancers. The lesion is commonly unilateral, but synchronous bilateral occurrences are seen in about 1% of cases, and metachronous bilateral occurrences are seen in about 12%–15% of cases.

The highest incidence of infiltrating ductal carcinoma is seen in patients aged 40–45 years. The incidence then declines for patients aged 45–50 years. Thereafter, the incidence increases with the age of the patient.

INFILTRATING LOBULAR CARCINOMA

Infiltrating lobular carcinoma accounts for 5%–15% of all breast cancers. It does not form a tumor until the disease is advanced. Even at that stage, the lesion manifests clinically as an ill-defined mass or thickening, similar to that found in fibrocystic changes of the breast (for example, epithelial hyperplasia). The difference is that infiltrating lobular carcinoma has a harder consistency.

Unless calcifications are associated with the disease, infiltrating lobular carcinoma does not have a characteristic mammography pattern. This situation further limits the early recognition of the lesion. The bilaterality and multicentricity of infiltrating lobular carcinoma are similar to those with LCIS: that is, 60% multicentric and 30% bilateral.

MUCINOUS CARCINOMA

Mucinous carcinomas are infiltrating, well-differentiated ductal carcinomas. They are also called "colloid carcinomas" or "gelatinous carcinomas." Mucinous carcinomas represent 1.5%–5% of all breast cancers. They occur more frequently in older women.

On physical examination, mucinous carcinomas are well-described tumors. However, because of the mucin content, the consistency is softer than that seen with other carcinomas. When the mucin content is high, the consistency will be soft and may mimic the consistency of the surrounding normal breast tissue. On mammography or ultrasonography, the image of the tumor is no different from that of other types of infiltrating carcinoma.

A mucinous tumor is slow growing, and, in general, has a better prognosis than a pure infiltrating ductal carcinoma.

MEDULLARY CARCINOMA

Medullary carcinoma accounts for 2%–7% of all invasive ductal carcinomas. The age incidence is 26–77 years, with a median age of 48 years.

On physical examination, a medullary carcinoma is a lobulated tumor, round, well circumscribed, soft, and possessing a relative mobility. Owing to these clinical characteristics, a medullary carcinoma is oftentimes mistaken for a fibroadenoma.

Medullary carcinoma has a better prognosis than does a high-grade infiltrating ductal carcinoma.

INFILTRATING PAPILLARY CARCINOMA

Infiltrating papillary carcinomas are rare. The highest incidence occurs at menopause (between ages of 60 years and 65 years), with a median age of 45 years.

On physical examination, invasive papillary carcinomas are firm to hard in consistency. The tumor size ranges from the microscopic to 3–4 cm.

Infiltrating papillary carcinomas are well-differentiated carcinomas; however, the prognosis for the patient is unfavorable.

TUBULAR CARCINOMA

Tubular carcinoma is a rare form of invasive breast cancer. Its incidence is 2%–4% of all breast cancers. It occurs mainly in patients in their mid forties, but has a range between 24 years and 80 years.

On physical examination, the tumor has poorly circumscribed borders. On palpation, it is firm to hard in consistency. The disease is frequently multicentric and bilateral.

On a mammogram, the tumor lacks a specific image. About 50% of cases of tubular carcinomas are associated with calcifications.

Tubular carcinoma is usually associated with a favorable prognosis.

BREAST CANCERS WITH UNUSUAL CLINICAL PRESENTATION

Two types of invasive carcinoma of the breast – Paget's disease of the nipple and inflammatory carcinoma – differ from the others because of their clinical presentation.

Paget Disease of the Nipple

Paget's disease of the nipple is not a special type of cancer. It is usually a DCIS that grows initially within the terminal ducts and then progresses by intraepidermal spread to the skin nipple.

CLINICAL PRESENTATION

At onset, Paget's disease of the nipple may be misdiagnosed as eczema. Its clinical course often reflects a long history of a combination of nipple symptoms – varying from an itching, burning sensation to oozing of a serous or serosanguineous secretion. If the disease remains unrecognized, it may progress until it takes on a variety of clinical appearances at the nipple skin, including redness, eczema, or ulceration.

Mammography does not contribute to the diagnosis.

Paget's disease of the nipple represents 1%–2% of breast cancers in women. In men, Paget's carcinoma is rare, with an incidence of less than 1% of all Paget carcinoma.

PHYSICAL EXAMINATION

In advanced cases, a palpable mass may be present. The figures that follow document the nipple changes that occur in patients with Paget's disease. The clinical and histopathologic features of the disease in men and in women is similar. (For an illustration of a male patient with Paget's disease of the nipple, see chapter 7, "Role of the Clinician – Male Breast," Figure 7.12.)

Figure 2.17
Figure 2.17 (A and B) shows the early clinical manifestation of Paget's disease of the nipple.

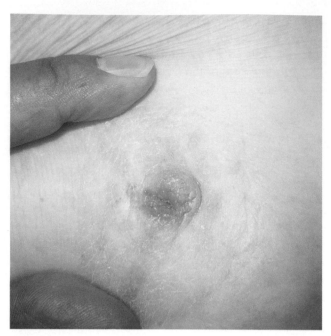

FIGURE 2.17A

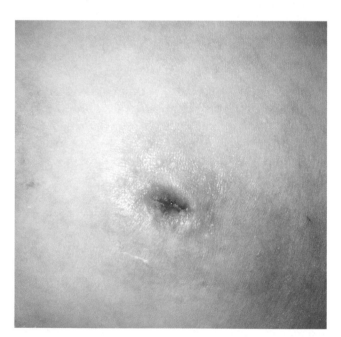

FIGURE 2.17B

Eczematous changes appear on the nipple skin, and the patient starts to experience some itchiness.

Figure 2.18

If Paget's disease goes unrecognized, redness of the nipple, with some erosion, edema, and wetness of the skin will appear [Figure 2.18 (A and B)]. Symptoms with this clinical presentation include skin itchiness and a burning sensation in the nipple area.

Figure 2.19

Figure 2.19 shows Paget's disease in a patient with inverted nipples. The patient's complaint was of local itchiness. The ulceration was hidden and could be noticed only when the skin of the nipple was separated.

Figure 2.20

The patient in Figure 2.20 had a more advanced case of Paget's disease. The nipple skin and the areo-

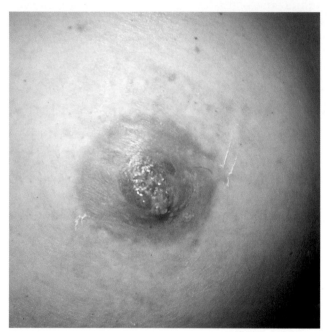

FIGURE 2.18A

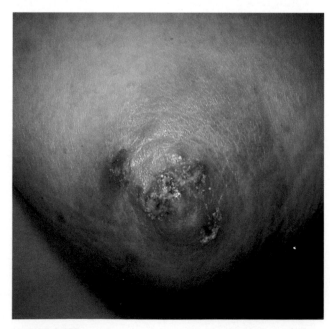

FIGURE 2.18B

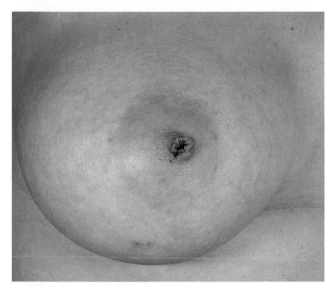

FIGURE 2.19

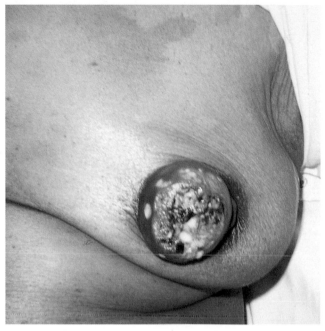

FIGURE 2.21

la are entirely invaded by the carcinoma. The skin has been replaced by granular tissue oozing serosanguineous fluid.

Figure 2.21
In Figure 2.21, the progression of advanced Paget's disease has completely destroyed the nipple–areola complex.

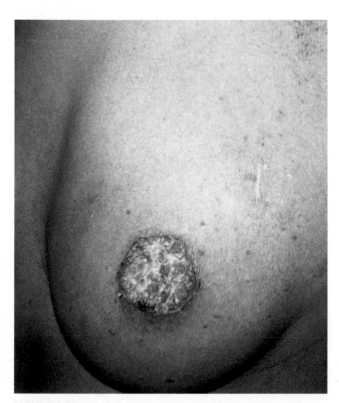

FIGURE 2.20

Both patients (Figures 2.20 and 2.21) had a large invasive carcinoma located central in the mid plane of the breast.

DIFFERENTIAL DIAGNOSIS

Several conditions affecting the nipple should be clinically differentiated from Paget's disease. These are: nipple adenoma, trauma, eczema and contact dermatitis.

With a nipple adenoma, the nipple is enlarged and occupied by the tumor. The skin is thin because of the distention produced by the tumor, but no ulceration is present.

Figures 2.22 and 2.23
Figure 2.22 shows a case of contact dermatitis of the areola skin. The nipple (arrow) showed no changes.

The patient in Figure 2.23 initially presented as a case of Paget's disease. The history described an oral trauma sustained a few days before the consultation. Edema, cellulitis, and oozing of the skin were present, but no ulceration was seen. Local treatment of the nipple resolved the problem.

Figures 2.24, 2.25, and 2.26
A biopsy of the skin nipple and adjacent ducts should be done to confirm a diagnosis of Paget's disease. The procedure usually takes place in an

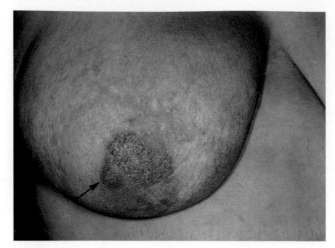

FIGURE 2.22

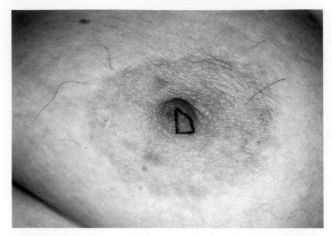

FIGURE 2.24A

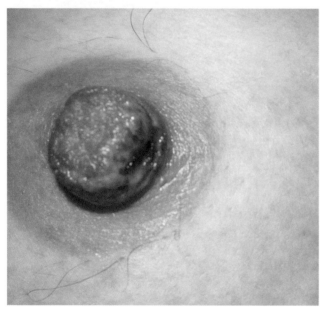

FIGURE 2.23

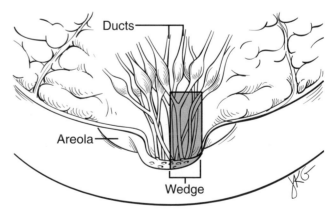

FIGURE 2.24B

ambulatory surgical facility. Local anesthesia and monitored intravenous sedation can be used. The skin is cleaned with antiseptic solution, and the area draped.

The skin incision is made in the shape of a wedge that extends to 25% of the nipple circumference [Figure 2.24 (A and B)]. The skin incision is then deepened to the area of the terminal ducts lying immediately behind the nipple (Figure 2.25).

Hemostasis should be thorough. In this area, the tissues are lax, and minimal bleeding may produce a large area of ecchymosis.

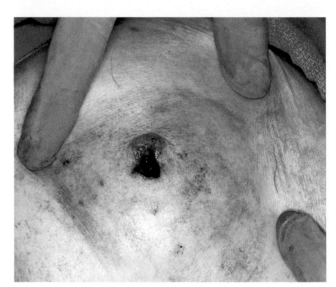

FIGURE 2.25

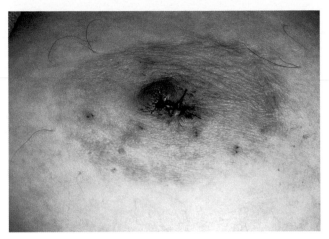

FIGURE 2.26

The skin approximation is carried out using #40 nylon sutures (Figure 2.26). This technique produces a good cosmetic result.

Figure 2.27

In this histopathology slide of a Paget's carcinoma (Figure 2.27), the Paget's cells are large, with pale cytoplasm and a large, prominent nucleus. (See also chapter 9, "Role of the Pathologist," Figures 9.104 and 9.105.)

Inflammatory Carcinoma

Inflammatory carcinoma of the breast is not a histologic type of cancer. It is the clinical presentation of the skin changes that occur when malignant cells permeate the lymphatic vessels within the subcutaneous tissue or dermis of the breast. The

prognosis for a patient with inflammatory carcinoma is poor.

CLINICAL PRESENTATION

Figures 2.28 and 2.29

Malignant cells permeate the lymphatic vessels of the subcutaneous tissue and dermis, obstructing lymph flow (Figure 2.28). Emboli of malignant cells within a lymph vessel cause the obstruction [Figure 2.29 (arrows)]. The obstruction causes the skin to become red and edematous, distending the pores. As the condition progresses, the patient starts to complain of a sensation of fullness in the breast.

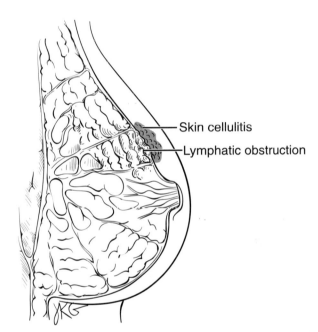

—Skin cellulitis
—Lymphatic obstruction

FIGURE 2.28

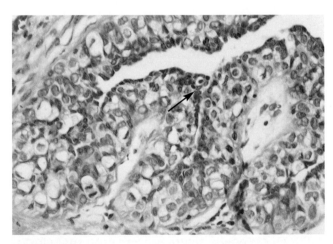

FIGURE 2.27

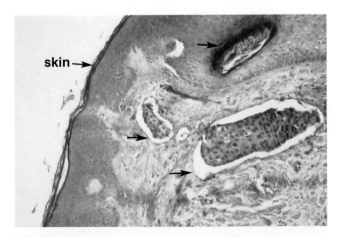

skin→

FIGURE 2.29

PHYSICAL EXAMINATION

Figure 2.30

The 35-year-old patient in Figure 2.30(A) had an aggressive infiltrating carcinoma of the right breast. The nipple was deviated lateral. There was some edema of the skin, as indicated by the indentation of the skin caused by the brassiere [Figure 2.30(A), arrow]. Pore dilatation was minimal.

The clinical diagnosis of inflammatory carcinoma was confirmed on surgical biopsy. The patient was treated with neoadjuvant chemotherapy to downstage the disease. A radical mastectomy with an immediate TRAM-flap breast reconstruction followed. (See chapter 13, "Role of the Plastic Surgeon," Figure 13.3.)

The degree of skin edema correlates with the size of the tumor. The patient shown in Figure 2.30(B) shows more pronounced edema. On physical examination, pressure applied to the skin leaves an indentation.

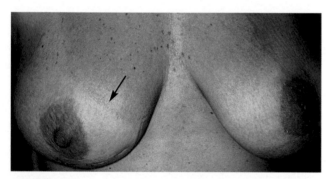

FIGURE 2.30A

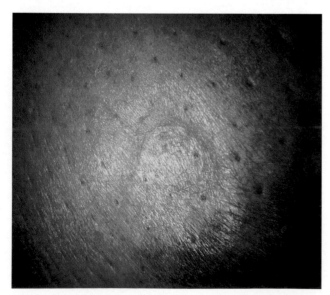

FIGURE 2.30B

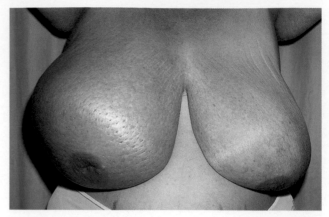

FIGURE 2.31

Figure 2.31

The 52-year-old woman shown in Figure 2.31 gave a history of progressive and rapid enlargement of the right breast. As the enlargement progressed, the patient started to complain of mastodynia. She also noted redness of the skin. No fever was present.

On physical examination, the breasts were asymmetrical. The right breast was enlarged, and on that side, the skin became erythematous, slightly warmer, and indurate. The skin edema distended the pores, producing the typical *peau d'orange* appearance commonly seen in inflammatory carcinoma.

On palpation, the entire breast was indurated. No defined tumor was palpable.

IMAGING

Figure 2.32

The mammogram of an inflammatory carcinoma is not specific (Figure 2.32). A diffuse increase in the density of the breast parenchyma occurs; but, in general, no defined tumor is seen. The skin is thickened owing to the edema. In this patient, the axillary node proved to be metastatic (arrow).

DIFFERENTIAL DIAGNOSIS

In its early stages, inflammatory carcinoma should be differentiated from duct ectasia, plasma cell mastitis, and breast abscess.

Duct ectasia is characterized by dilatation of the terminal breast ducts, accompanied by the presence of a thick fluid (resulting from the liquefaction of the desquamated cells – see chapter 4, "Symptoms of the Nipple–Areola Complex," Figure 4.22). Occasionally, acute exacerbation of a chronic state may manifest locally with a proliferation of

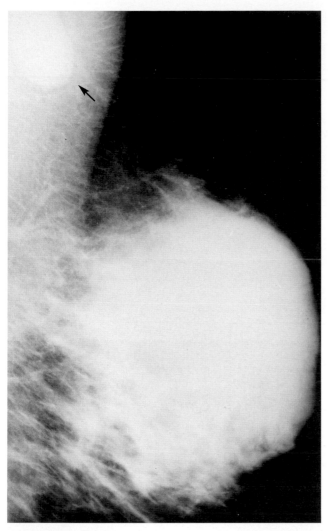

FIGURE 2.32

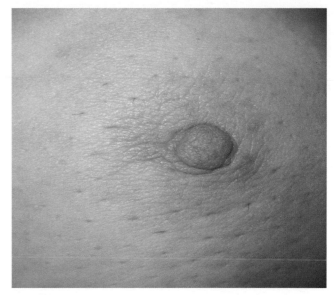

FIGURE 2.33

plasma cells around the ducts. If plasma cells are abundant, the overlying skin may develop cellulitis, sometimes accompanied by skin edema. A careful history, the symptom of warm skin, and resolution of the problem through the use of antibiotics make the differential diagnosis. If the skin symptoms persist for more than two weeks, an excisional biopsy is indicated.

Figure 2.33

Plasma cell mastitis (Figure 2.33) is often accompanied by a persistent burning sensation in the retroareolar region of the breast. The redness and edema of this condition are not as intense as in inflammatory carcinoma. The acute symptom subsides with antibiotics and the application of warm compresses.

A breast abscess differs from an inflammatory carcinoma in that the patient complains of pain and

may develop a fever. The skin is red and shiny, but the pores are not distended. The breast is tender.

A diagnosis of inflammatory carcinoma may be suspected from the clinical presentation and physical examination, but only the presence of malignant cells in the lymphatic vessels of the dermis make the diagnosis definite. (A finding of intratumoral lymphatic invasion is also considered to be an inflammatory carcinoma even in the absence of skin signs.) The surgical procedure can be done in an ambulatory surgical facility under local anesthesia and monitored intravenous sedation.

Figure 2.34

The biopsy should include an ellipse of skin that is removed in continuity with the underlying subcutaneous tissue and tumor. Figure 2.34 shows such an ellipse marked for incision.

Figure 2.35

As shown in Figure 2.35, the surgical specimen includes the dermis, the adjacent subcutaneous breast tissue and a segment of the tumor.

Figure 2.36

The histopathology diagnosis of inflammatory carcinoma should always be made from permanent rather than frozen sections, because failure to identify dermal involvement will inevitably lead to local recurrence in a patient initially treated with a mastectomy. The patient in Figure 2.36A had a modified radical mastectomy (left breast). Several months after surgery, she developed local recur-

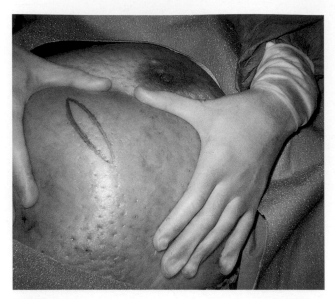

FIGURE 2.34

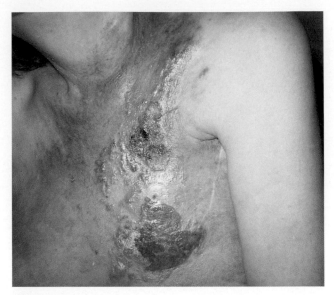

FIGURE 2.36A

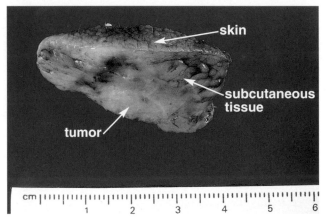

FIGURE 2.35

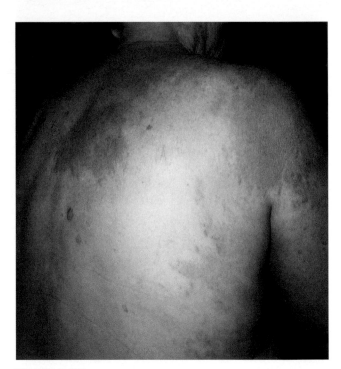

FIGURE 2.36B

rence on the skin. The skin involvement progressed rapidly, with spread to the skin of the right breast, the entire chest wall, and the back–the so-called carcinoma in cuiraiss (from the French, *cuiraisse* [shield] [Figure 2.36B]). Retrospective study of the permanent paraffin sections revealed malignant cells within the lymphatics of the dermis. Such cells had not been detected in the frozen diagnosis sections.

Patients with a confirmed diagnosis of inflammatory carcinoma should be treated with a few cycles of chemotherapy to downstage the disease before a mastectomy. An additional chemotherapy regimen should follow.

3

Pain

Mastodynia (breast pain) is the second most common breast symptom for which women seek a medical consultation. Because of the fear of breast cancer, mastodynia is a symptom of great concern to women. Although mastodynia is usually related to a benign condition, breast cancer may also manifest with pain as its initial symptom. Pain is reported to be associated with breast cancer in 8%–10% of all breast cancer cases.

OVERVIEW OF MASTODYNIA

Mastodynia can be cyclic or noncyclic.

Cyclic Mastodynia

Cyclic mastodynia is the most common type of breast pain. It is the result of water retention during the luteal phase of the menstrual cycle, which causes edema in the connective tissue. Characteristically, the pain is bilateral, occurs in the last two weeks of the cycle, and subsides at the start of menstruation.

In general, the severity of the symptom is related to the amount of swelling and the patient's threshold for pain. The pain is not actually localized; however, it frequently presents in the upper outer quadrant of the breast, which is the location of most of the breast parenchyma.

Cyclic pain – described as "heaviness," "aching," or "soreness" – is more common in women between the ages of 30 years and 35 years. Some patients may describe the pain as radiating toward the axilla and the inner surface of the arm, following the sensory branch distribution of the intercostal nerves.

Noncyclic Mastodynia

Noncyclic mastodynia is more localized than the cyclic type. It is usually unilateral. When the pain is related to an inflammatory process such as an abscess or plasma cell mastitis, it may be accompanied by local changes in the skin of the breast – redness, for example. It may also be accompanied by fever.

The most common causes of noncyclic mastodynia are mastitis and breast abscess, plasma cell mastitis, cyst, duct ectasia, and (occasionally) fibroadenoma and cancer.

Plasma cell mastitis – an acute exacerbation of chronic duct ectasia – may be accompanied by skin cellulitis and enlarged skin pores. (See chapter 5, "Skin Symptoms," Figure 5.11.) Fever is absent in plasma cell mastitis, but is usually present when the pain is related to an abscess or mastitis.

The pain associated with a macrocyst results from the sudden accumulation of fluid within the cyst cavity. Patients may describe the pain as "sharp," "dull," "fullness," or "a burning sensation." The burning sensation is due to irritation of the breast tissue caused by permeation of fluid through the cyst wall.

Duct ectasia occurs more frequently in menopausal and postmenopausal women. It is the result of glandular involution and secretory retention in the major ducts. The pain is usually felt in the periareolar region of the breast, and it may be accompanied by a thick, grumous discharge. (See "Fibrocystic Changes" in chapter 1, "Benign Tumors.")

For the most part, fibroadenomas and cancer are asymptomatic. The pain associated with these conditions is due to intratumoral hemorrhage, the extravasated blood causing intratumoral distention and pain.

REFERRED MASTODYNIA

In the absence of clinical or mammography findings, referred breast pain could be due to these conditions: intercostal neuralgia, Tietze's syndrome, *Herpes zoster*, or myalgia of the pectoralis muscle.

4

Symptoms of the Nipple–Areola Complex

The nipple–areola complex is the pigmented part of the skin that occupies the center of the anterior surface of the breast.

OVERVIEW OF AREOLA AND NIPPLE ANATOMY

The areola is the circular pigmented portion of the skin that surrounds the nipple. Its diameter averages 20–30 mm. Its color varies from pink or tan to dark brown, depending on the person's general coloring and, in the case of a woman, number of pregnancies. Darker color is seen in multiparous women owing to the melanocytic action of the pituitary gland during pregnancy.

The nipple is the cylindrical structure at the center of the areola. Its skin is irregular, rugged, and adherent to the adjacent tissue. When stimulated, the muscle fibers behind the skin cause the nipple to become erect. The anterior surface of the nipple has between eight and ten orifices. Each one receives a galactophorous duct (major duct).

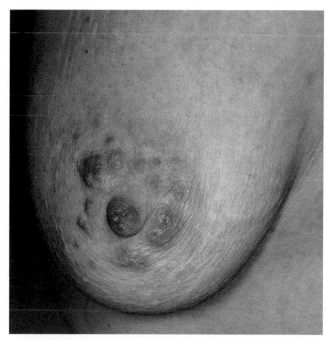

FIGURE 4.2

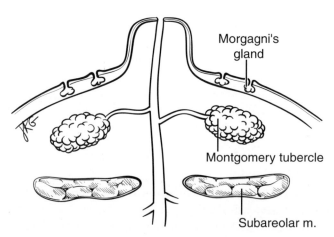

FIGURE 4.1

Figures 4.1 and 4.2

The skin of the areola is thin and adherent to the adjacent tissue planes. Small sebaceous glands called Morgagni's glands are found immediately beneath the skin of the areola in men and women alike (Figure 4.1). Morgagni's glands are connected to the exterior by skin pores. Their function is to lubricate the skin areola during nursing. Inconspicuous in the virginal breast, the nodules become apparent only when inflamed.

Deeper beneath the areola skin, muscle fibers keep the skin taut (Figure 4.1). At menopause, those muscle fibers lose their elasticity, and the areola becomes wrinkled.

Between the skin and muscle layers of the areola are the Montgomery tubercles (Figures 4.1 and 4.2). Montgomery tubercles lubricate the galactophorous

ducts during nursing. The glands are connected to the main ducts by small accessory ducts. As a result, they may become inflamed during pregnancy, after nursing or nipple manipulation.

Figure 4.3
Inflected Morgagni's gland in a male. If infected, the Morgagni's glands in the areola may form an abscess (Figure 4.3). Like any abscess, an abscess in a Morgagni's gland may drain spontaneously or may require incision and drainage.

NIPPLE SYMPTOMS

Several congenital anomalies of the nipple are possible. When nipples are absent, the condition is called athelia; when more than one nipple is present, the condition is called polythelia. (See chapter 6, "Role of the Clinician – Female Breast" [Figure 6.26B]).

The nipple can be the site of benign or malignant conditions. Among the benign conditions, fissures and mastitis are the most common. Fissures of the nipple and mastitis are most often seen during pregnancy and in nursing mothers. In pregnant or lactating women, a crack in the skin of the nipple is not an infrequent occurrence. The resulting fissure can be a point of bacterial entry.

Among the pathologic conditions that affect the nipple, the most common are nipple retraction or deviation, nipple ulceration, and nipple discharge. Nipple retraction and deviation are signs of advanced

breast carcinoma. Nipple ulceration may be the initial sign of Paget's disease. Nipple discharge is usually a sign of an underlying benign condition, such as an intraductal papilloma. However, it can also be a sign of an underlying carcinoma.

Nipple Retraction and Deviation

The nipple retraction phenomenon occurs when an infiltrating mass is located behind the nipple–areola complex and the fibrous tissue surrounding the terminal duct shortens as a result. Nipple deviation is usually caused by a large infiltrating mass located away from the nipple–areola complex. The deviated nipple always points toward the lesion. Both physical signs become more obvious in the inspection phase of the physical examination when the patient raises both arms overhead or presses both hands to hips (see chapter 6, Figures 6.2 and 6.3).

Nipple retraction and nipple deviation can be caused by benign or malignant conditions.

NIPPLE RETRACTION

When nipple retraction is caused by a carcinoma, a well-defined tumor is usually palpable behind the areola. The patient's history will reveal that the nipple has changed shape, having progressively been "drawing in." The patient may also state that she cannot "push it back out" (Figure 4.4). That is, nipple retraction caused by cancer cannot be everted.

Nipple retraction can also be caused by a chronic inflammatory condition such as chronic duct ectasia (Figure 4.5). In this case, no tumor is palpable. Rather, an elongated thickening that represents the chronically inflamed main terminal ducts is found. When the cause is an underlying benign condition such as chronic duct ectasia, the retracted nipple can be partially everted.

Nipple retraction should be distinguished from nipple inversion (Figure 4.6). Inversion is a congenital condition, present from the time of breast development. A good history will assist in making the differential diagnosis.

Mammography is usually nondiagnostic for duct ectasia. However, nipple retraction caused by carcinoma will image a stellate mass behind the nipple (see Figure 4.7).

Figure 4.4
Figure 4.4 shows the clinical presentation of the mammogram image illustrated in Figure 4.7. An infiltrating carcinoma located behind the nipple caused the retraction phenomenon.

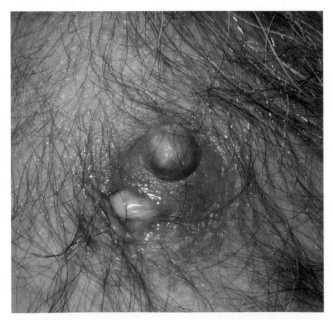

FIGURE 4.3

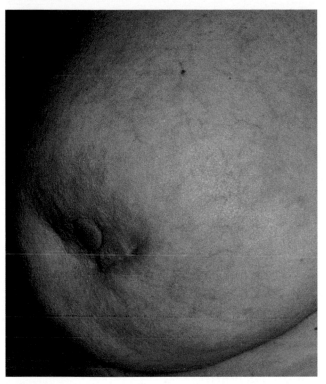

FIGURE 4.4

Figure 4.5

Figure 4.5 shows nipple retraction caused by chronic duct ectasia. The nipple can be partially everted when the areola adjacent to the nipple is squeezed. No tumor is palpable. The thickened duct feels wormlike. Bloodgood coined the term "variocele of the breast" for this condition.

Figure 4.6

Figure 4.6 shows the congenital condition of inverted nipple. When the areola is squeezed, the nipple can be easily everted.

Figure 4.7

A mediolateral oblique (MLO) mammogram for the patient shown in Figure 4.4 images a retroareolar mass. The mass measures approximately 1 cm in diameter and has long spicules extending into the surrounding parenchyma. The nipple is thickened because of tumor infiltration into the dermal lymphatic system, causing edema (arrow).

NIPPLE DEVIATION

A large malignant lesion that is located *away* from the nipple may cause nipple deviation.

Figure 4.8

The nipple deviation in Figure 4.8 is caused by a large infiltrating carcinoma located in the lower inner quadrant of the left breast (arrow). The sign became more apparent when, on inspection, the patient elevated her left arm. The skin adjacent to the mass was markedly dimpled.

Figure 4.9

The patient in Figure 4.9 had bilateral synchronous breast cancers. The mass in the left breast was located behind the nipple; the mass in the right breast

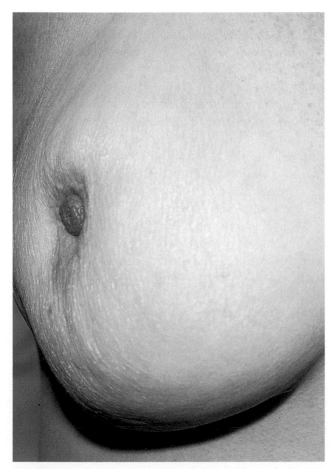

FIGURE 4.5

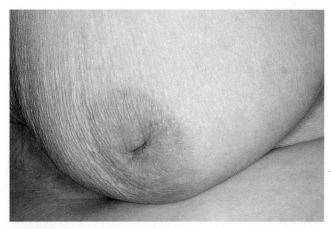

FIGURE 4.6

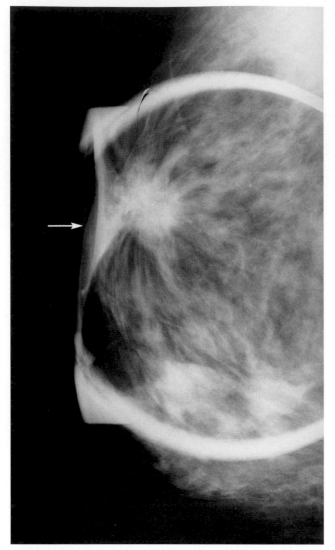

FIGURE 4.7

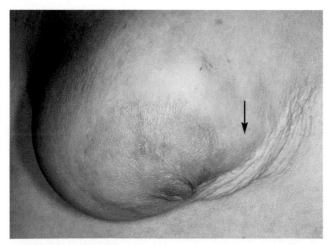

FIGURE 4.8

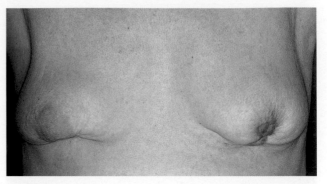

FIGURE 4.9

was located some distance away from the nipple. Both masses were hard in consistency with irregular borders, and both were fixed to the surrounding breast tissue. When the inspection was done with the patient's arms elevated overhead, the left nipple was retracted and the right nipple was deviated. These clinical signs alert the examiner to the location of the tumors.

Nipple Ulceration

Ulceration of the nipple skin should raise suspicion of Paget's disease, which, in its initial stage, might be mistaken for eczema of the nipple. When Paget's disease is the cause of nipple changes, the patient's complaint at onset is of an itching or burning sensation in the nipple area. The symptom is usually unilateral. Eczema of the areola is more often bilateral and symmetrical.

Paget's disease of the nipple is the clinical manifestation of ductal carcinoma in situ and/or invasive ductal of the terminal galactophorous ducts. Definitive diagnosis requires a biopsy of those ducts and the overlying skin to confirm the presence of Paget's cells in the skin layer of the nipple. (See chapter 2, "Malignant Tumors," [Figure 2.27]).

Nipple eczema may be the clinical manifestation of concomitant generalized eczema. If so, it is treated using the guidelines applicable to eczema elsewhere in the body.

Nipple Discharge

As a breast symptom, nipple discharge is most commonly seen in patients of perimenopausal age (40–45 years). It is the second most common breast symptom after a lump, and when bloody colored, it is one of the most alarming ones. However, nipple discharge is not a breast disease, but only a symptom. It may be caused by either a benign or a malignant process within the ducts.

NIPPLE DISCHARGE OVERVIEW

For all breast lesions, the incidence of associated nipple discharge is about 7%–10%. Of these, 10% are due to benign conditions, and approximately 3% are due to malignant ones.

The history for a patient with a nipple discharge should note

- the patient's age;
- whether the discharge is spontaneous or non-spontaneous, and if spontaneous, whether it is continuous or intermittent;
- whether the discharge issues through one or more nipple orifices;
- whether fever is present; and
- the physical characteristics (color, consistency) of the discharge.

When discharge is spontaneous, the patient will state that she noted a stain on her brassiere or nightgown, or that she noticed a discharge while showering (Figure 4.10). A non-spontaneous nipple discharge is one provoked by the patient or by the physician during physical examination (Figures 4.11 and 4.12). Of the two types, only spontaneous discharge has clinical significance.

Spontaneous nipple discharge that comes from only one nipple orifice is usually due to a pathologic condition such as an intraductal papilloma or a carcinoma. A non-spontaneous discharge usually issues through multiple nipple orifices and is always caused by a benign condition.

Certain medications such as the phenothiazines, tricyclic antidepressants, rauwolfia alkaloids, and methyldopa can cause a milky discharge (galactorrhea) either by increasing circulating prolactin, or by decreasing dopamine and stimulating serotonin at the hypothalamus. Oral contraceptives can also cause nipple discharge. In such cases, the color is milky with a grayish hue. A milky discharge may also be associated with endocrine syndromes that include amenorrhea – for example, Chiari–Frommel and Ahumada–del Castillo syndromes. (Readers may want to consult endocrinology and gynecology textbooks for more details.)

Fever may be present when the discharge is due to a retroareolar abscess that has spontaneously drained through the nipple or to puerperal mastitis.

Nipple discharge in a man – especially when that discharge is bloody – is significant because of its association with carcinoma.

Figure 4.10

In the case of spontaneous discharge shown in Figure 4.10, the patient related that she had noted a stain on her brassiere, and that the discharge had also occurred in the shower while cleaning the breast. Spontaneous discharge usually issues through only one nipple orifice, and is usually of a serous, sanguineous, or bloody color.

Figures 4.11 and 4.12

In Figures 4.11 and 4.12, cases of non-spontaneous nipple discharge become apparent only when the nipple is squeezed by the patient or by the physician during a breast examination. Non-spontaneous nipple discharge issues through multiple nipple orifices. The color of the discharge varies among white, gray, and green – singly or in combination. (Also see Figure 4.27.) Non-spontaneous discharge is a common symptom of duct ectasia; it may sometimes also occur without an underlying pathology.

Nipple discharges are classified as physiologic, pathologic, or false.

PHYSIOLOGIC DISCHARGE

Physiologic nipple discharge is seen in young patients during pregnancy or lactation, in patients

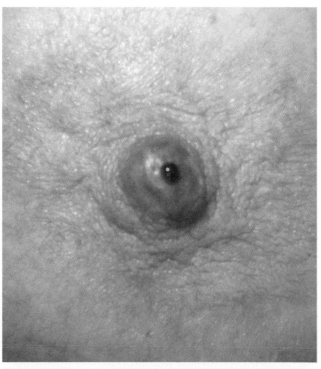

FIGURE 4.10

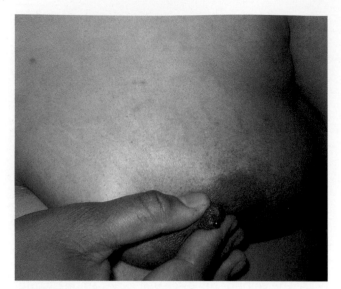

FIGURE 4.11

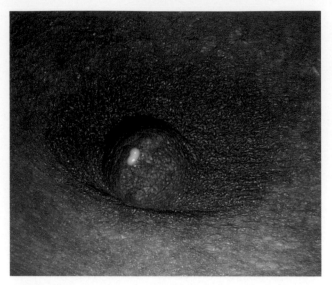

FIGURE 4.13

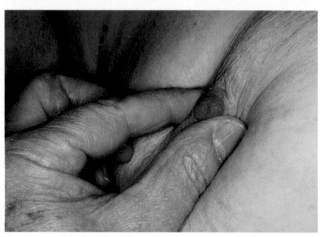

FIGURE 4.12

taking oral contraceptives, and in patients at peri-menopause or menopause.

Figure 4.13

In puerperal patients (Figure 4.13), milky discharge is physiologic. A thick, white discharge called colostrum may occur in the third trimester of pregnancy, just before the patient gives birth.

Owing to the dramatic decrease of estrogen and progesterone at the time of delivery, prolactin is re\leased by the pituitary gland and milk begins to be secreted. Suckling is the specific stimulus that maintains milk secretion. Suckling increases prolactin levels and induces the secretion of oxytocin in the posterior portion of the pituitary.

A milky discharge that persists for up to two years postpartum is not uncommon. Such a dis-

charge is still considered physiologic, and the patient need only receive an explanation and reassurance.

Milky discharge that persists for more than two years is called galactorrhea. Unlike a physiologic milky discharge, galactorrhea is usually bilateral and occasionally copious. The most common cause of galactorrhea is an increased level of prolactin, owing either to a pituitary tumor or to the administration of certain medications (tranquilizing agents, oral contraceptives, antihypertensives, and medications with direct action on the hypothalamus–pituitary axis, such as domperidone and metoclopramide). The differential diagnosis is made using the observation that galactorrhea induced by a pituitary tumor is usually accompanied by other endocrinologic symptoms such as amenorrhea and infertility, and that galactorrhea induced by medication becomes obvious from the patient's history.

Figure 4.14

Milky, grayish colored discharge is occasionally seen in patients at menarche (during the period of rapid breast development) or at menopause (Figure 4.14). Squeezing the nipples may provoke small quantities of the discharge, with a color varying from white to gray.

Figure 4.15

Bilateral milky discharge was seen in this patient who was taking oral contraceptives. In such patients, the discharge has a grayish hue.

Figure 4.16

Nipple discharge during pregnancy is not uncommon. The patient in Figure 4.16 is in the third trimester of her pregnancy.

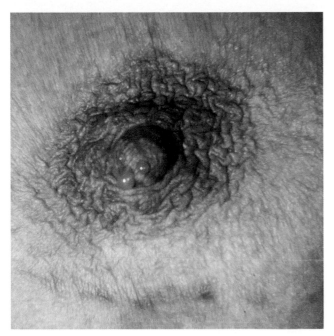

FIGURE 4.14

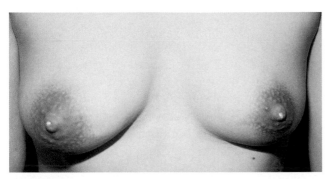

FIGURE 4.15

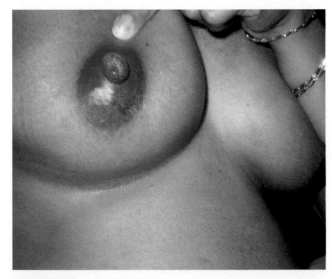

FIGURE 4.16

Discharge that occurs during pregnancy is usually bilateral and serosanguineous in color. It is due to epithelial proliferation and engorgement of the breast as the breast responds to the pregnancy.

Cytologic examination of this discharge may be misleading, because epithelial cells found in the smear could be interpreted as an intraductal papilloma. Intraductal papillomas and cancer are rare in this age group, and so cytology examination is not necessary. An explanation and reassurance are sufficient.

PATHOLOGIC DISCHARGE

Pathologic discharge is more common in patients at premenopausal or menopausal age. It is always spontaneous.

At the premenopausal age, intraductal papilloma (solitary or multiple) or intraductal papillomatosis is usually the underlying cause. However, the author has seen this type of lesion in patients below the age of 20, and in one patient that was an octogenarian.

Duct ectasia, which manifests with a thick, "sticky" discharge, is commonly see at the paramenopausal age.

At menopause or post menopause, cancer – associated with a serous, sanguineous, or bloody discharge – is usually the underlying cause.

Purulent discharge is usually due to the spontaneous drainage of a breast abscess through the duct system.

Figure 4.17

Solitary papillomas like the one shown in Figure 4.17 (arrow) are rare. They are usually located at the end of the milk duct sinus, and they have a narrow, fragile stalk containing capillaries.

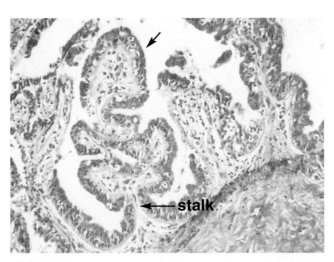

FIGURE 4.17

Minimal trauma or torsion to the fibrovascular stalk may cause bleeding. When a certain amount of blood accumulates within the duct, the lesion will manifest clinically as a spontaneous discharge.

Nipple discharge that issues through only one nipple orifice is usually caused by an intraductal papilloma.

Figure 4.18

Multiple papillomas, as shown in Figure 4.18, are more common than solitary papillomas. Multiple papillomas are also multicentric. The bleeding mechanism is similar to that for solitary papillomas.

Solitary and multiple papillomas are both microscopic; on clinical examination no tumor is palpable. Papillomas cannot be imaged using mammography or ultrasonography. The diagnosis is therefore usually made on clinical grounds: that is, spontaneous discharge (serous, sanguineous, or bloody), issuing through only one nipple orifice.

Figure 4.19

The 50-year-old patient in Figure 4.19 complained chiefly of a spontaneous bloody discharge. The discharge issued through only one orifice. Adjacent to the areola, a 2-cm, hard, irregular tumor with serrated borders was found. Pressure over the tumor also produced the discharge. Macroscopic tumors that are associated with a nipple discharge of a bloody and serous or watery color are usually papillary carcinomas.

Figure 4.20

The thick, non-spontaneous, yellow-colored discharge demonstrated in Figure 4.20 is characteristic

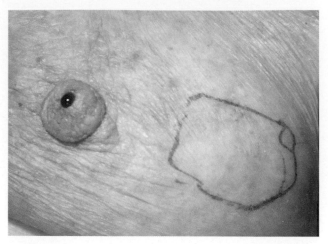

FIGURE 4.19

in patients that have duct ectasia. The discharge may be unilateral or bilateral.

Duct ectasia is a type of fibrocystic change in the breast (see chapter 1, "Benign Tumors"). It occurs mostly in premenopausal patients as a result of the hormone imbalance that occurs at that time. As a result of the hormonal changes, desquamation of cells from the duct wall and increased secretion within the ducts occur. The secretion becomes stagnant and accumulates within the duct lumen, distending the duct. Eventually, the patient starts to complain of breast "fullness" and a burning sensation in the nipple area that may radiate centrifugally to other quadrants of the breast. This symptom induces the patient to squeeze the nipple and produce the thick discharge.

Nipple discharge resulting from duct ectasia is non-spontaneous. The color varies from white, gray,

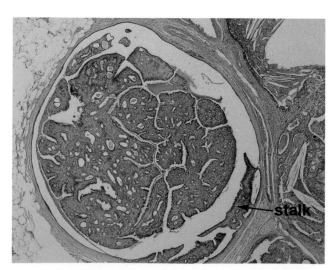

FIGURE 4.18

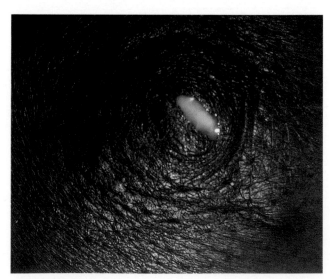

FIGURE 4.20

and brown in the acute phase to a yellow-orange color as the process becomes chronic.

Figures 4.21 and 4.22

The histopathology slide of duct ectasia in Figure 4.21 shows dilatation of the affected terminal ducts with an intraluminal secretion resulting from cellular debris. Inflammatory cells surround the duct, causing periductal inflammation.

With time, the duct wall becomes thin, dilates, and adheres to the areola skin. If the duct is close to the areola skin, a fistula may develop in the adhered area (Figure 4.22).

Figure 4.23

The patient shown in Figure 4.23 complained of episodes of progressive mastodynia unrelated to the menstrual cycle. The pain was always accompanied

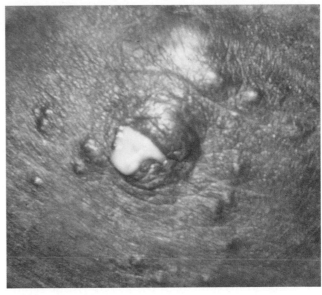

FIGURE 4.23

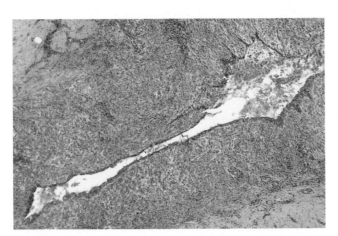

FIGURE 4.21

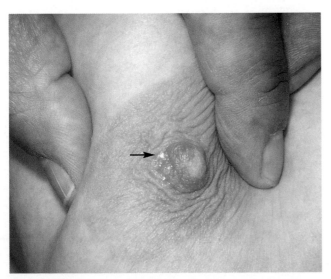

FIGURE 4.22

by fever, which subsided after the discharge had occurred. Purulent nipple discharge of this kind is usually due to spontaneous drainage of a breast abscess through the duct system.

The patient was treated with antibiotics. When the acute symptoms subsided, the central ducts were excised. (See chapter 11, "Surgical Treatment of Benign Breast Lesions.")

FALSE DISCHARGE

False nipple discharge is discharge in the area of the nipple–areola complex that does not issue through a nipple orifice (Figure 4.22, arrow). The most common conditions that can mimic nipple discharge are inverted nipple, trauma, eczematous lesions, and infected Montgomery gland cysts with fistulas. False nipple discharge may also be seen in patients with advanced Paget's disease or trauma to the nipple (see chapter 2, "Malignant Tumors").

Patients with inverted nipples may complain that "something is coming out of the nipples." This comment is a reference to the sebum-like secretion from the sebaceous glands located within the invaginated skin. This secretion (which usually is thick) sometimes forms a crust. During the examination, the examiner should try to clean the skin surface from which the secretion issues. Careful observation will demonstrate that the secretion does not issue through a nipple orifice. Cleansing the skin with the nipple everted takes care of the problem and rules out an underlying skin lesion such as Paget's disease.

PHYSICAL EXAMINATION IN CASES OF NIPPLE DISCHARGE

Physical examination of the nipple–areola complex is part of a general examination of the breast, which is described in detail in chapter 6, "Role of the Clinician – Female Breast." In the present section, the emphasis is on a physical examination when nipple discharge is the patient's presenting symptom.

As always, an inspection should be done with the patient in the sitting position. During the inspection, notice should be given to any skin changes in the nipple–areola complex – for example, prominent Montgomery gland cysts; nipple inversion, retraction, deviation, or ulceration; and crust, exudate, or spontaneous nipple discharge.

Palpation is done with the patient in the supine position. Because intraductal papillomas and ductal papillomatosis (the lesions that usually cause pathologic nipple discharges) are both typically microscopic, a tumor is seldom palpable in patients with nipple discharge. In such cases, the examiner can use two maneuvers – bimanual compression of the breast (Figure 4.24) and digital pressure around the areola (Figure 4.25) – to assist in determining which sector of the breast holds the underlying pathology.

Macroscopic papillomas are soft. They can sometimes be missed during palpation because their consistency may be softer than that of the adjacent breast parenchyma. However, if the palpation is gentle (no hard pressure on the breast), the examiner may be able to detect them.

Figures 4.24 and 4.25

In the bimanual compression maneuver (Figure 4.24), the examiner presses gently but firmly down against the chest wall, starting from the area of the nipple–areola complex and working outward (arrows). Nipple discharge that becomes evident with bimanual compression and comes out through several nipple orifices indicates a benign process, commonly duct ectasia.

In the digital palpation maneuver (Figure 4.25), the examiner uses the index finger of the dominant hand to palpate the nipple–areola complex. The palpation starts approximately 2 cm from the margin of the areola and moves radially toward the nipple. The palpation should be done firmly and slowly, starting at the 12 o'clock radius and proceeding systematically clockwise until the circle is complete. The pressure point that elicits a discharge indicates the sector in which the pathology is located. A discharge that

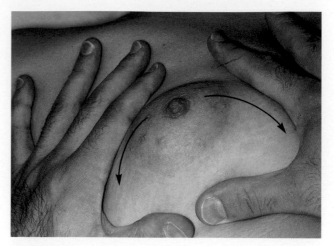

FIGURE 4.24

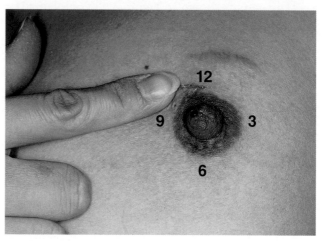

FIGURE 4.25

issues through only one nipple orifice is usually related to a papilloma or cancer.

Figures 4.26 through 4.31

When nipple discharge is elicited in a physical examination, the characteristics of the discharge – color, consistency, and whether the discharge issues through one or several nipple openings – should be noted.

The consistency of the discharge can be thin or thick, sticky or not.

The color of the discharge varies with the underlying pathology. The author has been able to document seven different color types: milky, multicolored, purulent, serous, serosanguineous, bloody, and watery (no color).

Milky discharge (Figure 4.26) is a physiologic discharge and may persist for up to two years postpartum.

White, gray, or multicolored nipple discharge is always non-spontaneous. It is commonly seen in duct ectasia. When duct ectasia is the underlying pathology,

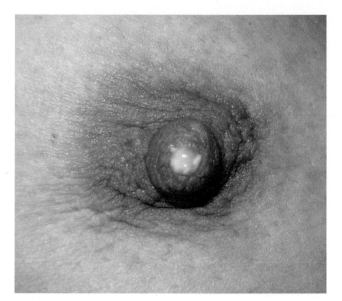

FIGURE 4.26

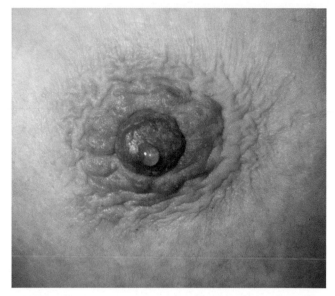

FIGURE 4.28

the discharge issues through several nipple orifices and is grumous (sticky) on palpation (Figure 4.27). The patient requires no treatment, excepting reassurance.

The serous (Figure 4.28), serosanguineous (Figure 4.29), bloody (Figure 4.30), and watery (Figure 4.31) types of nipple discharge are most often attributable to a benign condition (most commonly intraductal papillomas).

The age incidence of serous, serosanguineous, and bloody discharge is the fourth decade; however, those types of nipple discharge have been reported in patients in their early twenties and in octogenarian patients. A serous discharge, especially if dark-

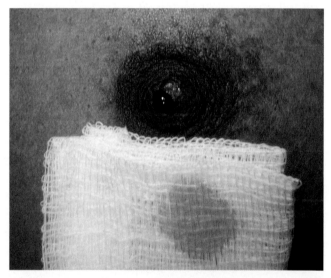

FIGURE 4.29

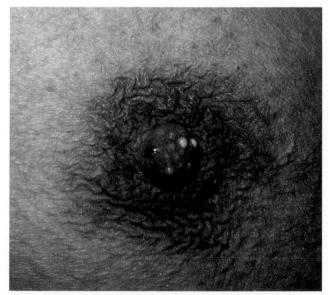

FIGURE 4.27

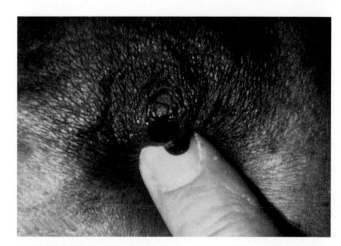

FIGURE 4.30

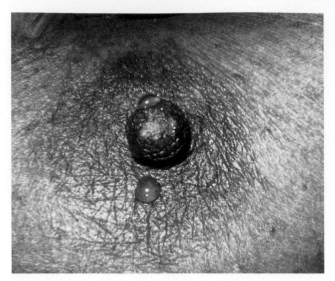

FIGURE 4.31

colored, may appear bloody at inspection. A simple test such as applying a gauze pad against the discharge may indicate whether blood is present (Figure 4.29). *The gauze test should not replace the guaiac test.*

Watery discharge (Figure 4.31) has no color. Although watery discharge is the least common type of nipple discharge, it is the type more often associated with carcinoma.

Figure 4.32
Nipple discharge in a male patient is rare. When present, such discharge should always raise suspicion

of a malignancy. The man in Figure 4.32 presented with a serous discharge issuing through one orifice of the left nipple.

TREATMENT

Galactorrhea is a physiologic discharge and requires no treatment. If, however, it persists for more than two years postpartum, an investigation must be undertaken to rule out pituitary adenoma.

Duct ectasia requires no surgical treatment. The patient should be reassured and advised to refrain from manual manipulation (which has a "suckling" effect that will prolong the symptom).

Spontaneous nipple discharge – especially of the serous, serosanguineous, bloody, or watery type – must be investigated. Investigation is required even if a mammogram is negative or a smear reports negative cytology. If the underlying pathology is macroscopic and localized, then only the involved sector of the breast is excised. The excision should include an ample margin of normal breast tissue.

Intraductal papillomas and ductal papillomatosis are usually microscopic, multiple, and multicentric. The most effective surgical treatment is excision of the terminal major ducts – the breast site where these lesions are usually located. For patients under the age of 30 years (or older, but anxious to have children and nurse), the removal of a single duct or the segments containing the pathology may be the preferred choice. The surgical technique is discussed in chapter 11, "Surgical Treatment of Benign Breast Lesions."

Figure 4.33
The specimen in Figure 4.33 comes from a patient operated on for a bloody nipple discharge. The

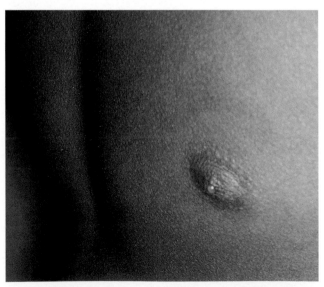

FIGURE 4.32

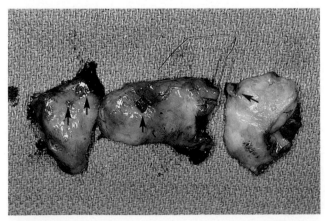

FIGURE 4.33

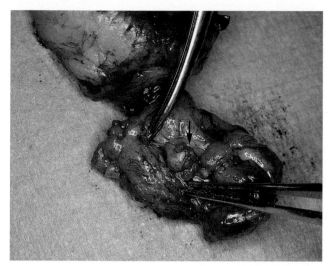

FIGURE 4.34

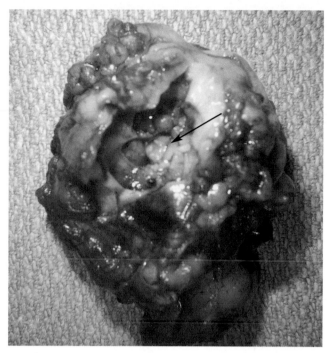

FIGURE 4.36

gross specimen was opened along the path of a dilated duct. Four macroscopic papillomas (arrows) are present.

Figure 4.34

Figure 4.34 shows the gross specimen of a patient operated on for a bloody nipple discharge. The dilated duct has been opened to show the papilloma (arrow). The lesion was soft and not palpable. Often, a large papilloma can not be distinguished in consistency from the surrounding breast tissue.

Figures 4.35 and 4.36

The chief complaint of the 49-year-old patient in Figure 4.35 was of intermittent spontaneous watery (no color) discharge from the right nipple. She described the discharge as "water colored," and each

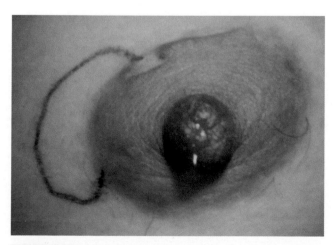

FIGURE 4.35

time she pressed around the nipple, "liquid shot out like water." Palpation located a mass just lateral to the areola margin at the 9 o'clock position. The mass measured 4 cm in diameter. It was hard, with irregular borders. Pressure applied to the mass produced a projectile colorless discharge.

Watery nipple discharge is rare. When present, it may be associated with a malignant process 50% of the time. In this patient, the lesion was an intracystic papillary carcinoma (arrow).

Figure 4.36 shows the gross specimen from the same patient. The specimen has been opened to show the large papillary carcinoma (arrow).

Figures 4.37 and 4.38

Although nipple discharge is often caused by microscopic tumors that cannot be imaged during mammography or ultrasonography, large papillomas may be imaged as denser soft tissue, even without the use of contrast material. The author has been able to document several cases.

Figure 4.37 is the mammogram of a patient with an intraductal papilloma in the retroareolar region. It images as a lobulated 1-cm × 1-cm mass with a surrounding lucency (arrows).

Figure 4.38 is a sonogram from the same patient. Although mammography imaged only one papilloma, the sonogram imaged multiple papillomas as

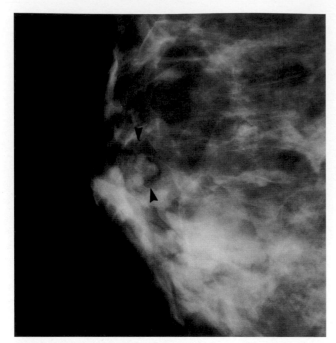

FIGURE 4.37

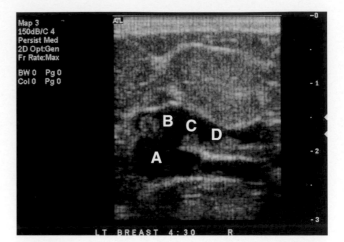

FIGURE 4.38

small mural nodules (B), (C), (D) within a dilated, fluid-filled duct (A).

Figures 4.39

Gallactography may assist in diagnosing large papillomas or papillary carcinomas when they image as a filling defect within a duct. The galactogram in Figure 4.39 is from a patient with chronic duct ectasia. It images dilated subareolar ducts, with normal peripheral arborization of the ducts. The arrows point to the dilated portion of the ducts and to the normal arborization of some ducts.

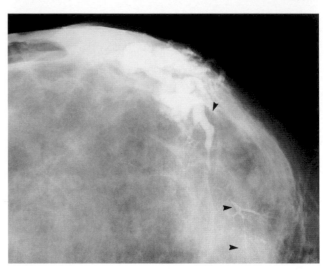

FIGURE 4.39

5

Skin Symptoms

The skin of the breast can be the localized site of a primary breast problem or a local manifestation of a generalized skin disorder. For the latter, readers should consult the appropriate dermatology textbooks.

Skin changes on the breast may or may not be related to intrinsic breast pathology.

SKIN CHANGES UNRELATED TO BREAST PARENCHYMA PATHOLOGY

The most common benign conditions of the breast skin that the author has encountered more frequently in medical practice are ecchymosis, *Herpes zoster,* hemangioma, and Mondor's disease.

Ecchymosis

Ecchymosis of the breast skin may occur in patients who are taking anticoagulant medication or who have sustained trauma to the breast.

Figure 5.1
The patient in Figure 5.1 had been taking a warfarin sodium medication for a long time.

Figure 5.2
The patient in Figure 5.2 had been involved in a car accident as a passenger. She was wearing her seat belt. An area of ecchymosis developed on the right breast at the 3 o'clock radius. She also had a small tender mass in this area.

When an ecchymosis is due to trauma, finding a mass at the site of the injury is not uncommon. The mass may be soft if it occurs immediately or hard if it develops late. A mass that presents immediately after an accident commonly represents a hematoma. A mass that develops a few weeks or months after an injury represents fat necrosis. The extravasated blood reacts with the fat of the subcutaneous adipose tissue, which becomes gelatinized, forming the mass. With time, the mass becomes hard and irregular – to the extent that it may mimic a carcinoma. A careful history will resolve the differential diagnosis between carcinoma and fat necrosis.

Figure 5.3
A fine-needle aspiration biopsy and a mammogram may assist in making the determination between

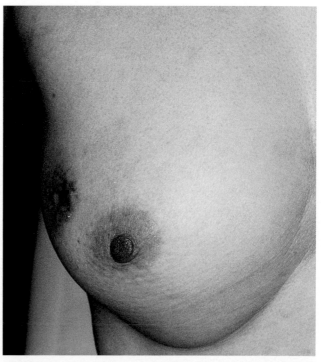

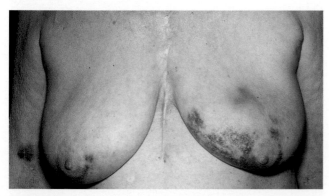

FIGURE 5.1

FIGURE 5.2

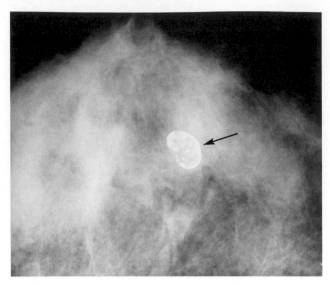

FIGURE 5.3

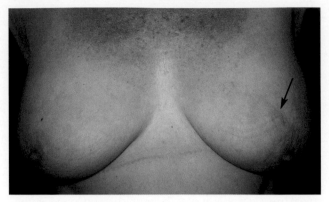

FIGURE 5.5

a carcinoma and fat necrosis. A mammogram will image a well-defined mass as an "oil cyst." An oil cyst is lucent, with a well-defined capsule (Figure 5.3), a radiographic finding that is diagnostic of fat necrosis. (See also Figure 8.11 "Role of The Radiologist.")

Herpes zoster

A *Herpes zoster* infection is of viral origin. It affects nerve dermatomes. Clinically, it presents with severe pain, followed 2–3 weeks later (the incubation period) by the appearance of vesicles on the skin of the breast. The process is self-limiting, and treatment is symptomatic.

Figure 5.4

This vesicles of *Herpes zoster* are characteristic, being arranged linearly following the track of the affected skin dermatomes.

Hemangioma

Figure 5.5

Hemangiomas in the skin or subcutaneous tissue are recognizable from the bluish purple discoloration (arrow) and "spongy" consistency of the skin. In large hemangiomas, a bruit may be present.

Figure 5.6

A mammogram may image a hemangioma. The mediolateral oblique (MLO) projection in Figure 5.6 demonstrates rounded densities within the mid portion of the left breast. These densities have the appearance of phleboliths or granulomas. Several of the densities have lucent centers. In the presence of skin

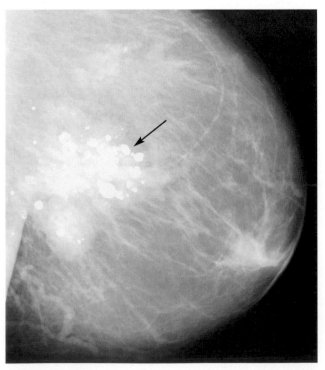

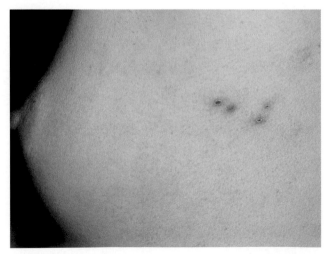

FIGURE 5.4

FIGURE 5.6

hemangioma, this finding presents as hemangioma within the breast, because the patient had no history of injected silicone.

Mondor's Disease

Mondor disease bears the name of the French surgeon who first described it in the breast. The condition is an inflammation of a superficial vein in the breast (usually the thoracoepigastric vein).

The thoracoepigastric vein extends from the inguinal area, ascending along the abdominal wall to the lower costal margin, the breast, and the axilla, to become a tributary of the axillary vein. Inflammation can occur in any portion of its trajectory.

The pain that a patient with Mondor's disease experiences is self-limiting. It requires only symptomatic treatment (or no treatment at all). The "cord" typically disappears within a few weeks to a few months.

Figure 5.7

Trauma is usually responsible for the inflammation of Mondor's disease. Often, the patient does not recall the injury. She becomes aware of the condition only when she notices a thick "cord" in the skin area over-

lying the affected vein (arrow). The redness and pain usually subside in a few days. The vein becomes thrombotic and, on palpation, feels "cord-like."

Figure 5.8

Mondor's disease may be also be seen postoperatively following breast surgery. In such instances, the cause of the inflammation and thrombosis is the trauma caused by the needle traversing a vein in the subcutaneous tissue (arrow).

The thoracoepigastric vein can also be traumatized in the process of an axillary dissection. Inflammation of the vein may then propagate to the brachial vein. The postoperative development of a "cord-like" structure in the inner surface of the arm is not an uncommon occurrence, following a mastectomy. The patient should receive an explanation and reassurance.

SKIN CHANGES RELATED TO BREAST PARENCHYMA PATHOLOGY

Breast disease, benign or malignant, may be associated with skin changes. Intrinsic breast pathology

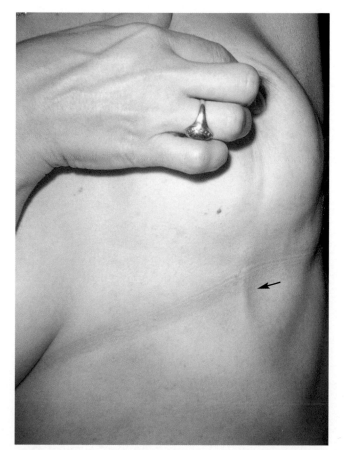

FIGURE 5.7

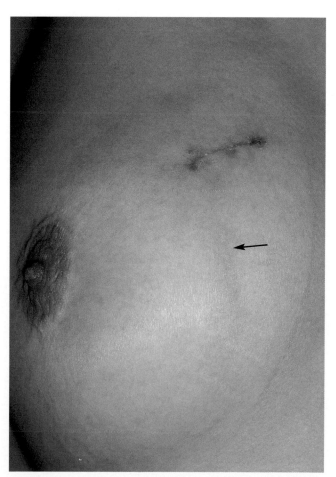

FIGURE 5.8

that causes changes in the breast skin is usually malignant. With earlier detection of breast cancer, skin changes are now seen less frequently.

The skin changes that most commonly occur in breast cancer are redness, edema, dimpling, and ulceration.

Redness and Edema

Skin cellulitis and edema are seen in breast infections (puerperal patients), in duct ectasia, in plasma cell mastitis, and in inflammatory carcinoma.

Figure 5.9

Figure 5.9 shows a case of puerperal mastitis with lymphangitic spread.

Breast infections are seen most often in the early stages of lactation – so-called puerperal mastitis. The pathogen usually enters at the nipple. If the infection is not attended to, it propagates centrifugally through the ducts to the breast parenchyma. Progression of the inflammatory process may lead to formation of an abscess. This complication should be suspected when the patient develops pain and fever, and the skin of the breast becomes edematous.

Antibiotics and local application of heat may resolve the problem.

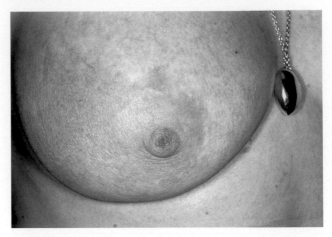

FIGURE 5.10

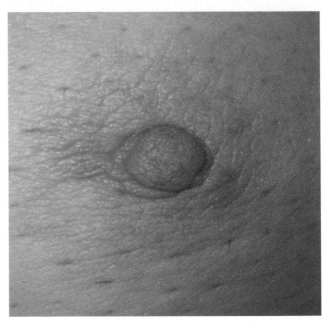

FIGURE 5.11

Figures 5.10 and 5.11

Plasma cell mastitis, a form of fibrocystic change in the breast, may also present clinically with redness of the skin and enlarged pores (Figure 5.10), symptoms that mimic inflammatory carcinoma. If the condition is plasma cell mastitis rather than inflammatory carcinoma, the symptoms should subside with antibiotic treatment. Persistent or increasing skin cellulitis intractable to a course of antibiotics should raise suspicion of an inflammatory carcinoma. If two weeks of conservative treatment produce no change in the symptoms, a biopsy should be done. The biopsy should include the skin, the subcutaneous tissue, and a portion of the adjacent breast tissue to clarify the diagnosis. (See chapter 2, "Malignant Tumors," Figure 2.35.)

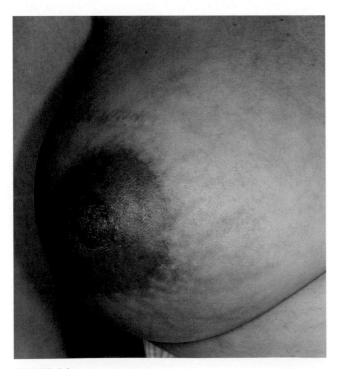

FIGURE 5.9

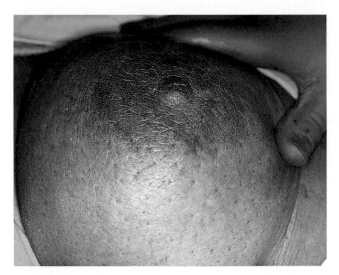

FIGURE 5.12

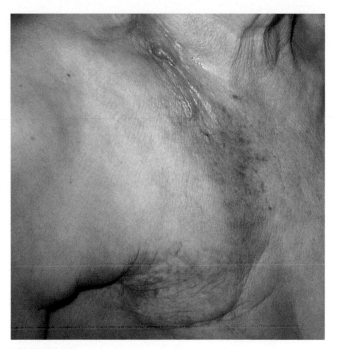

FIGURE 5.14

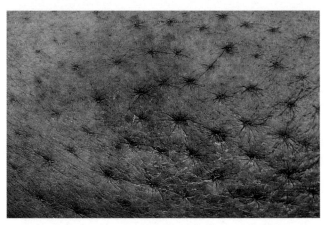

FIGURE 5.13

Figures 5.12 and 5.13

Skin redness accompanied by edema and enlarged skin pores is usually the clinical manifestation of an inflammatory carcinoma (Figure 5.12). The edema and distended pores are the result of retrograde flow from lymphatics blocked by emboli of malignant cells (see chapter 2, "Malignant Tumors," Figure 2.29).

In the patient in Figure 5.13, the tumor was large and occupied almost the entire breast. The skin is edematous and the pores are enlarged, giving the appearance of orange peel *(peau d'orange)*.

Figure 5.14

Figure 5.14 shows skin cellulitis in a patient who was treated with a modified radical mastectomy. Two years after the surgical procedure, this woman developed cellulitis of the skin on the ipsilateral side. The cellulitis commenced at the innermost site of the scar

and extended upward, along the lateral border of the sternum, reaching the area of the neck. Histopathology confirmed a clinical diagnosis of recurrent carcinoma. Retrospective review of the mastectomy histopathology specimen slides revealed intratumoral lymphatic spread.

Figure 5.15

The patient in Figure 5.15 had a large mass that occupied the retroareolar area of the left breast. The mass extended to the medial quadrants. The patient consulted when she noticed the skin changes (redness and edema) on the left breast. A clinical diagnosis of inflammatory carcinoma was confirmed by the histopathology: tumor cells were identified in the dermal lymphatics.

Treatment planning for inflammatory carcinoma must await the permanent-section diagnosis. This patient was treated initially with four cycles of chemotherapy to downstage the disease. A modified radical mastectomy and additional chemotherapy followed. She also received tamoxifen and radiation to the chest wall.

Skin Dimpling

Skin dimpling is usually a physical sign of locally advanced carcinoma. The dimpling is caused by a shortening of the Cooper's ligaments as they become involved with the carcinoma.

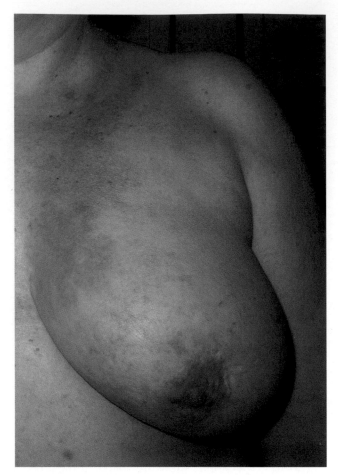

FIGURE 5.15

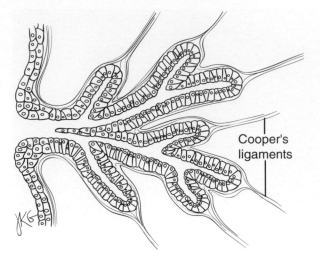

FIGURE 5.16

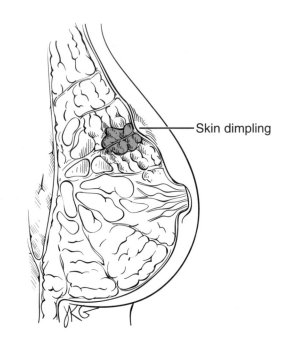

FIGURE 5.17

Figures 5.16 and 5.17

Cooper's ligaments are the suspensory ligaments of the breast; they support the breast tissue to the skin. The relationship that the ligaments have with the skin can be best understood through the embryology (Figure 5.16).

By the end of the third month of gestation, squamous cells from the surface of the skin begin to invaginate to form the nipple bud. As the invagination continues, primary lobules and ducts develop. Eventually, the invagination carries a layer of the superficial fascia inward. That layer becomes the Cooper's ligaments.

The fibroconnective tissues of the Cooper's ligaments extend through the breast as a network and attach to the skin. If a tumor invades the ligaments, the skin retracts (Figure 5.17) and the skin dimples.

Figures 5.18 and 5.19

Often, skin dimpling can be detected upon simple inspection. Having a patient elevate her arms or press hands to hips may bring the examiner's attention to a problem that is not evident when the inspection is done with the arms at the side (Figure 5.18).

A mammogram in the cranial-caudal (CC) Figure 5.19 view shows a tumor in the mid-lateral quadrant. The mammogram images the tumor and the prominent Cooper's ligaments involved with the invasion (small arrow). The skin dimpling is also imaged (large arrow).

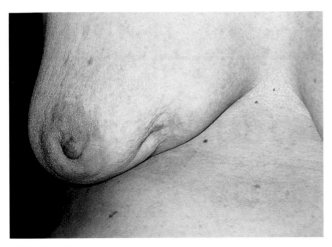

FIGURE 5.18

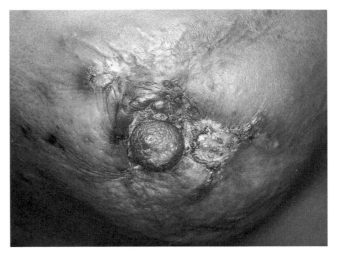

FIGURE 5.20

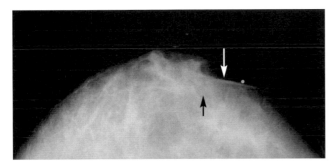

FIGURE 5.19

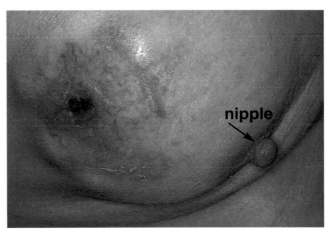

FIGURE 5.21

Skin Ulceration

Skin ulceration that it is caused by a locally advanced carcinoma is a clinical sign of inoperability.

Figure 5.20
The patient in Figure 5.20 had a large carcinoma located in the retroareolar area. It was locally advanced, with multiple satellite skin nodules. Some of the nodules exhibit impending ulceration. The cellulitis around the ulcerated area is due to inflammation around the exposed cancer.

Figure 5.21
Figure 5.21 shows a locally advanced carcinoma with ulceration of the skin. The tumor occupies both lateral quadrants. The skin is purplish colored, owing to compression of the capillaries of the adjacent skin by the large tumor. The ulceration reflects direct invasion of the skin and is not attributable to a lack of blood supply. The telangiectactic changes around the ulcerated skin are a sign of a late carcinoma.

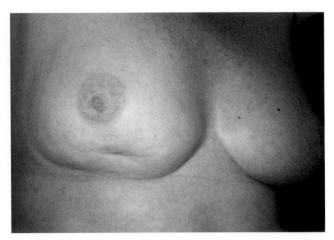

FIGURE 6.12

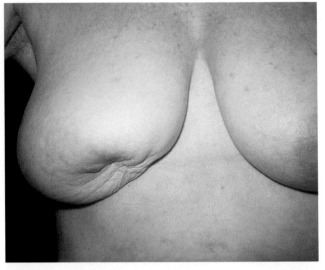

FIGURE 6.14

Figure 6.13

In Figure 6.13, during a "hands on hips" portion of an inspection, a loss of contour is seen in the left breast just above the areola, the site of a tumor. Nipple retraction is also present.

Figure 6.14

An inspection with the patient pressing hands to hips (Figure 6.14) demonstrates a cancer behind the areola at the 6 o'clock radius. The nipple is flattened and pulled inward. It points down, toward the lesion. An area of skin dimpling is also seen.

The degree of nipple retraction and associated skin dimpling depends on the size of the tumor. The larger the lesion, the more pronounced the associated skin dimpling.

Figures 6.15, 6.16, and 6.17

Asymmetry and loss of breast contour can be a normal finding, but it can also be observed with large

benign tumors – for example, giant fibroadenomas or phyllodes tumors.

In Figure 6.15, inspection of a patient with "hands on hips" shows loss of contour for the left breast owing to a locally advanced carcinoma (arrow).

In Figure 6.16, the inspection shows loss of contour and symmetry for the left breast owing to a tumor that extends from the retroareolar area into both upper quadrants. The physical findings became more prominent when the patient pressed hands to hips or raised her arms overhead.

Figure 6.17 shows marked dimpling of the skin owing to a large carcinoma located in the lower inner quadrant of the left breast. Although the skin dimpling in this patient was obvious even with direct inspection, the physical sign became more pronounced as the patient pressed hands to hips. The

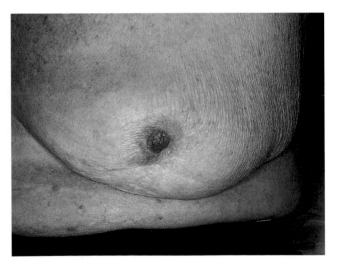

FIGURE 6.13

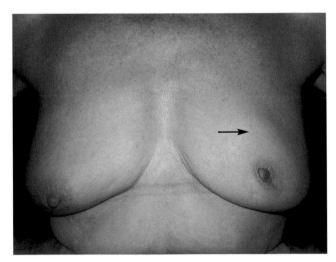

FIGURE 6.15

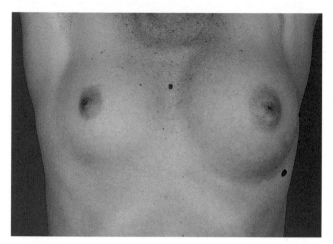

FIGURE 6.16

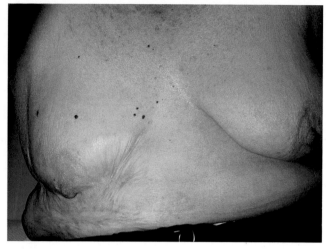

FIGURE 6.19

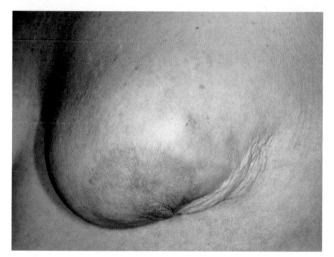

FIGURE 6.17

Figure 6.18

Nipple inversion should not be mistaken for nipple retraction. A careful history will reveal that the nipple has been inverted for many years, usually from puberty. Pressing around the areola or nipple with the index finger and thumb should easily evert an inverted nipple. Also, an inverted nipple is not thickened (as is usual in the case of a carcinoma).

Figure 6.19

Several years before the examination shown here, the patient in Figure 6.19 had suffered a third-degree burn resulting in nipple deviation and skin changes. A careful history helped to make a differential diagnosis.

Figure 6.20

There is always an impulse on the part of the physician to examine first the area of skin dimpling

nipple is deviated, and it is pointing toward the lesion. Note that an infiltrating carcinoma located behind the nipple causes nipple retraction, but one located away from the nipple area causes nipple deviation.

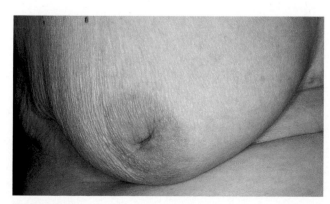

FIGURE 6.18

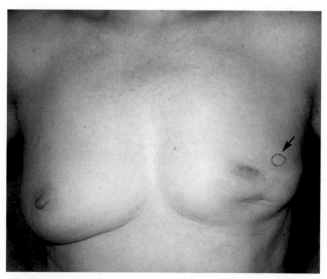

FIGURE 6.20

and to persevere in trying to find a lesion at that site. But the area of skin dimpling may not necessarily correspond to the tumor location.

In the patient shown in Figure 6.20, a retraction phenomenon manifested as skin dimpling in the lower quadrant of the left breast in the midline. A carcinoma was located in the upper outer quadrant (arrow).

SKIN CHANGES

Skin abnormalities such as a change in color (erythema) may be present in patients with acute mastitis or breast abscess. When a benign disease such as plasma cell mastitis causes cellulitis, the skin is smooth and warm. When an abscess causes cellulitis, the skin may be warmer and tender. In neither condition are the skin pores enlarged. Cellulitis, edema, and enlarged skin pores (the so-called *peau d'orange* appearance) are the clinical findings of an inflammatory carcinoma. (See chapter 2, "Malignant Tumors," Figures 2.30B and 2.31.)

Figure 6.21

The 36-year-old patient in Figure 6.21 was one year postpartum. She complained of progressive enlargement and redness of the right breast. A large tumor was present in the lower outer quadrant of the right breast just beneath the areolar margin (arrow). When the inspection was done with the patient's arms raised, the nipple deviated downward, pointing toward the site of the tumor. A clinical diagnosis of inflammatory carcinoma was confirmed by an incisional biopsy of the tumor and overlying skin. (See chapter 2, "Malignant Tumors," Figure 2.35.)

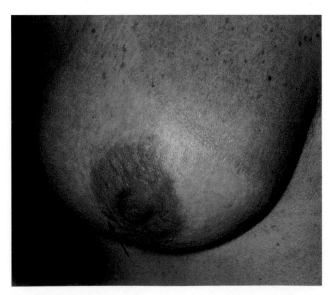

FIGURE 6.21

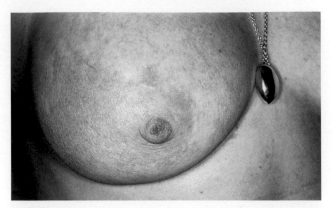

FIGURE 6.22

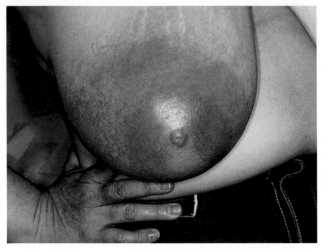

FIGURE 6.23

Figures 6.22 and 6.23

The patients in Figures 6.22 and 6.23 each had skin cellulitis caused by a benign condition. For the patient in Figure 6.22, the cellulitis was the result of acute exacerbation of chronic duct ectasia. The patient in Figure 6.23 had an acute retroareolar abscess.

NIPPLE SKIN AND NIPPLE–AREOLA COMPLEX

The size and color of the areola and nipple vary among women. In nulliparous women, the color of the areola is pinkish; the color darkens after the first pregnancy and lactation.

The skin of the nipple–areola complex can be the site of various pathologic entities, benign or malignant. The most common are enlarged Montgomery or Morgagni glands, cysts, congenital inverted nipples (with or without crusty discharge), nipple retraction and deviation, nipple discharge, and Paget's disease. (See chapter 4, "Symptoms of the Nipple–Areola Complex.")

Congenital anomalies of the breast and nipple documented here include supernumerary breast, supernumerary nipple (polythelia), amastia (absence of the breast), and hypoplastic breast.

Figure 6.24

Embryologically, the mammary gland forms within a ventral epidermal ridge known as the "milk line." By the sixth week of human development, the milk line appears as a bilateral thickening of the ectoderm that extends from the axilla to the inner aspect of the thigh.

Along this line, the embryo has approximately 10–12 pairs of breasts. Except for the breast pair located in the developing thorax (Pair IV, the normal pair), the other pairs involute.

Failure of the embryo's superfluous breast pairs to involute is responsible for certain congenital abnormalities, the most common of which are accessory breast tissue (supernumerary breasts) and supernumerary nipples (polythelia).

Figures 6.25 and 6.26

Supernumerary breasts typically develop from breast pair I, II, or III. Usually, they are not fully de-

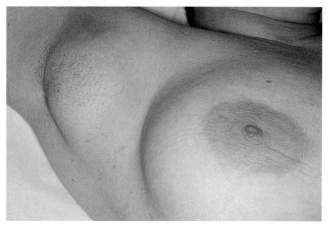

FIGURE 6.25

veloped; they lack an areola or nipple, or both. The most frequent site of a supernumerary breast is the axilla (pair II, Figure 6.25).

Small supernumerary breasts are asymptomatic and should be left alone. But large supernumerary breasts – such as that shown in Figure 6.25, which caused discomfort to the patient when the arm was adducted – should be treated. Such a problem is normally the only indication for surgery. However, the author has also documented a fully developed supernumerary breast within a breast (vestige from pair III) that was excised for cosmetic reasons (Figure 6.26A).

The incidence of benign and malignant tumors in a supernumerary breast is equal to that of the fully developed breast.

Supernumerary nipples (Figure 6.26B) may develop in either sex and at any location along the milk line, from the clavicle to the inguinal region. However, they are more commonly seen under the surface of the breast mount or on the upper abdomen (pairs V–VII).

When rudimentary, an ectopic nipple may be mistaken for a pigmented nevus.

Figure 6.27

The congenital absence of a breast and nipple is termed "amastia." When the breast tissue is absent but the nipple has developed, the condition is called "amazia." Amastia or amazia associated with a congenital absence of the pectoralis major muscle and syndactyly characterize Poland's syndrome.

Amastia is a rare condition thought to be due to a complete involution failure.

In the neonatal period, breast enlargement is the result of transplacental estrogen stimulation and is therefore physiologic. Acquired amastia is the result

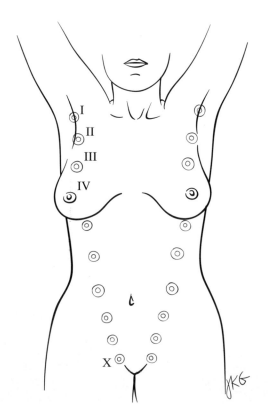

FIGURE 6.24

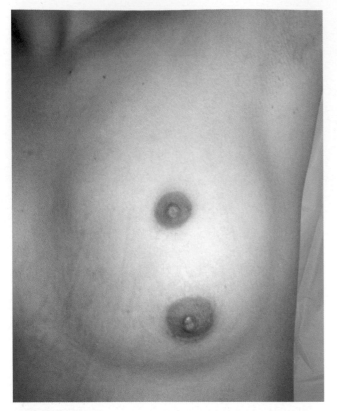

FIGURE 6.26A

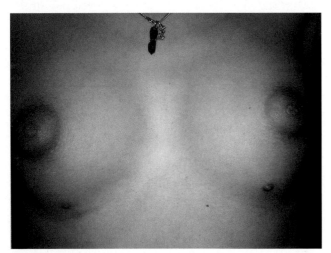

FIGURE 6.26B

when an unaware surgeon fails to recognize this condition, mistaking it for a "tumor."

In the patient in Figure 6.27, the breast parenchyma and pectoralis muscle are absent and only the nipple remains (Poland's syndrome).

Figure 6.28
The condition of having an underdeveloped breast is called hypoplasia. Figure 6.28 shows a pa-

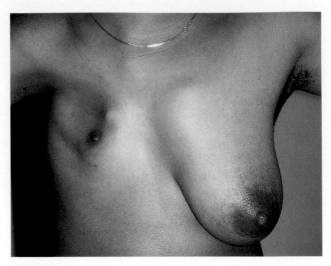

FIGURE 6.27

tient whose left breast failed to fully develop. No tumor or mass was palpable. The mammogram and sonogram were normal. For psychological reasons, the patient had an augmentation mammoplasty. Cosmetic surgery should be delayed until the patient reaches the age of 18–20 years, by which time the gland is fully developed.

Examination of the Supraclavicular and Infraclavicular Areas

While the patient is still in the sitting position, examination of the axilla and the supraclavicular area should follow the inspection.

Good access to the supraclavicular area can be obtained by having the patient bring her shoulders forward while she presses hands to hips. With this maneuver, the posterior cervical triangle hollows, facilitating examination of the neck.

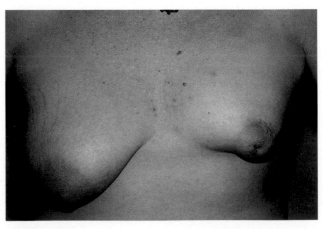

FIGURE 6.28

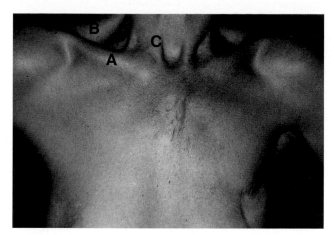

FIGURE 6.29

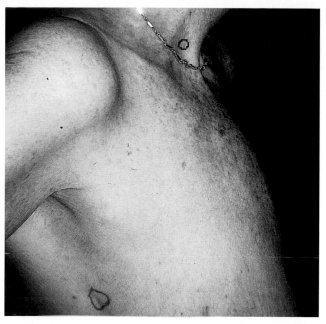

FIGURE 6.31

The anterior and posterior triangles of the neck should both be examined.

Figure 6.29

The posterior triangle of the neck (Figure 6.29) is delimited anteriorly by the external border of the sternocleidomastoid muscle (C), inferiorly by the clavicle (A), and posteriorly by the anterior border of the trapezius muscle (B). The anterior triangle of the neck is delimited posteriorly by the sternocleidomastoid muscle, anteriorly by the lateral border of the trachea, and by the sternoclavicular junction.

Although the supraclavicular nodes are located near the angle of the clavicle and the suprasternal notch, the examination should extend medially and laterally from the junction of the manubrium of the sternum along the superior border of the clavicle toward the anterior border of the deltoid muscle.

Figure 6.30

The examiner palpates the supraclavicular area while standing in front of or behind the patient. The author finds the latter position easier (Figure 6.30).

Figure 6.31

Although breast cancer infrequently metastasizes to the lymph nodes on the anterior triangle of the neck, that area should also be included in the examination. The patient in Figure 6.31 had bilateral mastectomies. In a follow-up examination, a large metastatic cervical node was detected in the anterior triangle of the neck. Metastatic residual axillary node was also detected along the anterior axillary line.

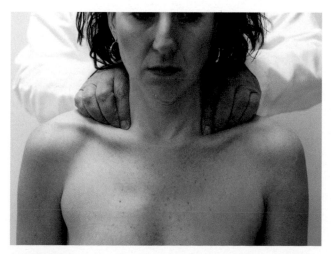

FIGURE 6.30

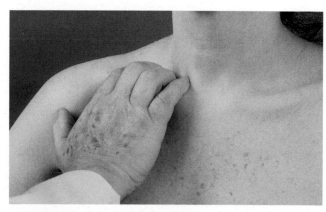

FIGURE 6.32

Figure 6.32

The infraclavicular area should also be palpated while the patient is still in the sitting position. The patient's arms should be at her side. The examiner should feel for the clavicle and travel down along its anterior surface to "fall" in the costal plane (Figure 6.32). Palpable infraclavicular nodes are a poor prognostic sign given their location behind the pectoralis major muscle.

Examination of the Axillae

Because the clinical staging of breast cancer is based in great part on the axillary findings, a thorough examination of the axilla is an important part of a breast examination.

Anatomically, the axilla is a potential space in the shape of a pyramid – with four walls, a base, and an apex. The anterior wall is the pectoralis major muscle, the posterior wall is the latissimus dorsi muscle, the medial wall is the chest wall, and the lateral wall is the head of the humerus. The costoclavicular junction is the apex. (See Figure 12.29 in chapter 12, "Surgical Treatment of Malignant Breast Lesions.")

Figure 6.33

To carry out the examination, the physician should stand to the patient's side, on the side of the axilla being examined. For best access to the axilla, the pectoralis major muscle should be relaxed. To achieve the necessary relaxation, the examiner should hold the patient's ipsilateral arm slightly flexed at the elbow while the patient elevates the arm toward forehead level. The examiner then introduces his or her fingers toward the apex of the axilla and against the chest wall. At the same time, the examiner brings the pa-

tient's arm over, to rest on the examiner's arm (Figure 6.33). This maneuver not only relaxes the pectoralis major muscle, but also allows the examiner to bring fingers high toward the vertex of the axilla.

The palpation should be gentle. Unless metastatic, lymph nodes are soft. Pressing hard against the chest wall will compress the nodes, and the examiner may miss them.

Examination begins at the most apical portion of the axilla and continues down and against the chest wall. Upon completion of the maneuver, the examiner's hand should be supinated, and, from that position, the examiner can palpate the posterior surface of the pectoralis major muscle, where the lateral axillary and Rotter's nodes are located.

If nodes are found, their consistency and their mobility should be noted. Non-pathologic nodes are mobile and soft; metastatic nodes are large and harder. As metastasis within a node progresses and fully replaces normal tissue, it perforates the node's capsule. At that point, the node may become fixed.

The examination of the axilla is also a good opportunity to examine the axillary extension of the breast (tail of Spence).

Bimanual Palpation of the Breast

Regular palpation of the breast is done in the supine position, after examination of the axillae. But while the patient is still in the sitting position, the examiner should bimanually palpate the breast to assess the texture and consistency of the breast tissue.

Figures 6.34 and 6.35

As the term implies, bimanual palpation uses both of the examiner's hands. The lower hand supports the breast ridge, and the upper hand gently palpates the entire breast by pressing against the lower hand (Figure 6.34). The examiner must not "pinch" the breast (Figure 6.35), because that technique gives a false sensation of a mass or tumor that should be avoided.

Breast consistency varies from patient to patient. Consistency is firmer in premenopausal patients in whom fibrous tissue dominates. The atrophic tissue of a postmenopausal patient is "granular," the "granules" representing the atrophic breast tissue surrounded by fat.

Examination in the Supine Position

The last phase of a breast examination is palpation with the patient lying in the supine position. This

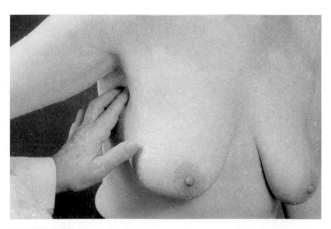

FIGURE 6.33

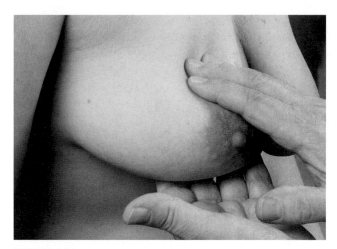

FIGURE 6.34

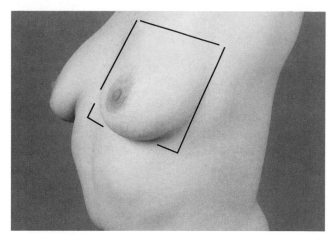

FIGURE 6.36A

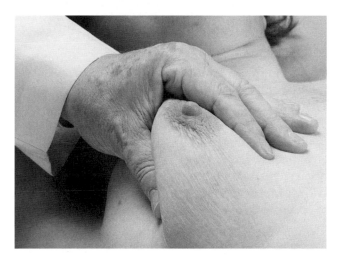

FIGURE 6.35

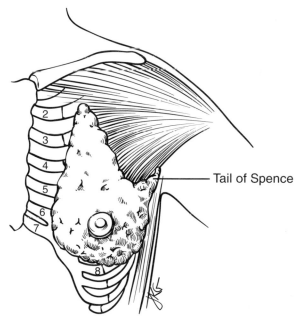

FIGURE 6.36B

palpation uses the tips of the fingers to press the breast against the chest wall. The technique should be gentle and systematic, covering the entire breast surface. As stated by Bloodgood, the examiner should palpate as if "playing the piano" – meaning gentle palpation with all the fingers oscillating, as if touching a piano keyboard.

Each quadrant of the breast should be examined separately.

Figure 6.36A and 6.36B

Anatomically, the breast tissues extend from the second to the seventh (or sometimes the eighth) rib, and from the lateral border of the sternum medially to the lateral border of the latissimus dorsi muscle laterally. The breast also extends to the axilla as a "tail" called the tail of Spence. Occasionally, it extends toward the xiphoid or the rectus fascia area (or both). Breast palpation should include all of these areas.

A small pillow should be placed under the patient's back on the side being examined, and the patient's ipsilateral arm should be raised above her head. This shifts the breast medially, flattening it over the anterior thoracic wall.

Figure 6.37A and 6.37B

Figure 6.37 illustrates examination of the right breast. To facilitate the examination and to make it more comfortable for the examiner, he or she should stand on the patient's right side when palpating the medial quadrants of the right breast and on the patient's left side when palpating the lateral quadrants of the right breast. Each quadrant – medial and lateral – should be examined separately.

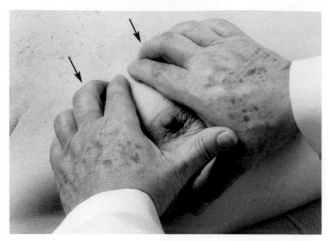

FIGURE 6.37A

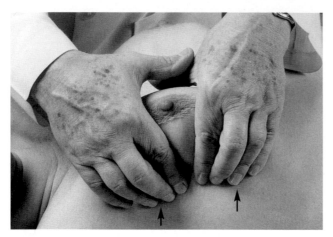

FIGURE 6.37B

Palpation of the medial quadrants starts at the sternum at the level of the second rib and progresses toward the midline (A). In this fashion, the palpation proceeds downward toward the breast ridge (inferior portion of the breast).

The palpation should be bimanual, using the tips of the fingers. As the palpation progresses downward, the left hand will palpate the segment already palpated by the right hand.

The palpation of the lateral quadrants extends from the border of the latissimus dorsi muscle to the midline of the breast (B). It starts at the level of the axilla (tail of Spence) and finishes at the breast ridge. Again, as the examination progresses downward, the right hand overlaps the examination already done with the left hand.

It should be emphasized that three areas of the breast are commonly thicker than the others. One is in the tail of the breast; another is the area of the breast ridge; and the third is the subareolar area.

The most common physical findings during breast palpation are nodules, masses, and tumors. When a lesion is found, or when an area of the breast feels different from the rest of the gland, that lesion or area should be studied more thoroughly.

NODULES

Nodules are the most common finding during breast palpation. They are the clinical presentation of the fibrocystic changes that occur in the female breast from menarche to menopause. (See "Fibrocystic Changes" in chapter 1, "Benign Tumors.")

Nodules are small, non-tender lesions that may be localized in only one portion of the breast or (more commonly) scattered throughout the gland. The clinical presentation can be unilateral or bilateral.

Nodule size varies according to the phase of the patient's menstrual cycle at the time of the examination. The nodules are finer and more pronounced at the end of the cycle; they should not be mistaken for the false "nodularities" present in a post-menopausal woman's breast. The "nodules" palpated in the breast of a postmenopausal patient actually represent fat lobules of the subcutaneous layer encircled by Cooper's ligaments and atrophic breast tissue. The differential diagnosis is made using the knowledge that "false nodules" are larger, more circumscribed, and softer than the true nodules found in younger patients.

Figure 6.38

Figure 6.38 shows a specimen containing small cysts. The consistency of small cysts depends on the

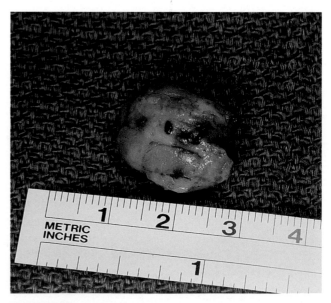

FIGURE 6.38

amount of fluid that they contain. When the fluid is under tension, the cysts feel hard. When the cysts are numerous, palpation produces an irregularly "bumpy" sensation similar to that felt when touching a surface made up of small pebbles or sliding the fingers over green peas or chickpeas resting on a flat surface.

MASSES OR TUMORS

The terms "mass" and "tumor" are used indiscriminately, a fact that often confuses not only patients but also physicians. Because the management of a mass differs from the management of a tumor, it becomes important to differentiate these lesions.

A tumor is a clinical entity that has three dimensions: width, height, and depth.

An example of a tumor is the palpatory finding of a fibroadenoma (see chapter 1, "Benign Tumors," Figure 1.6). On palpation, the examiner will feel only the most superficial part of the tumor and its edge; but, using stereotactic sense, he or she will perceive that something is "behind" that surface.

A mass differs from a tumor in that it is bi-dimensional, having only width and length. It actually represents an area of indurated breast tissue. During palpation, a mass is elongated rather than round. It gradually blends with the adjacent breast tissue and has no well-defined border. A mass is the most common clinical sign found in fibrocystic changes such as adenosis and hyperplasia.

Differential Diagnosis on Palpation

When an area of the breast feels different from the rest of the gland, that finding should be further studied in an attempt to make a clinical differential diagnosis. The examiner should take note of the area's delineation, size, consistency, mobility, and attachment or fixation.

DELINEATION

Benign and malignant tumors are both ovoid or round. The former have well-delineated margins; the margins of the latter are irregular. A benign tumor typically has a smooth surface; however, some fibroadenomas – although well delineated – may have a lobulated surface.

The degree of lobulation in a tumor depends on how much cellular proliferation is being contained by the surrounding fibrous tissue. (See chapter 1, "Benign Timors," Figures 1.3 and 1.4). Lobulation should not be mistaken for the irregular border of a malignant tumor.

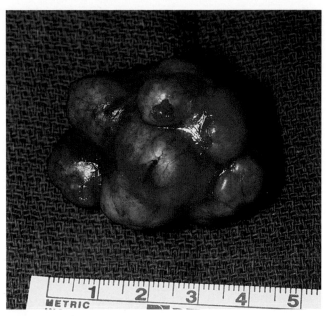

FIGURE 6.39

Figure 6.39
Figure 6.39 shows the multilobulated but smooth surface of a phyllodes tumor. The lobulations result from proliferating cells being entrapped within fibrous tissue. The consistency is firm.

Figure 6.40
The surface of the carcinoma in Figure 6.40 is well delineated, but irregular and hard.

SIZE

The size of a tumor should be noted in centimeters, and not compared to objects such as eggs, grapes, or walnuts.

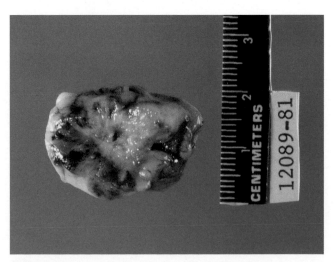

FIGURE 6.40

Tumor size does not indicate whether a tumor is benign or malignant. Fibroadenomas may attain a large size, especially when they change into giant fibroadenomas or phyllodes tumors. A large malignant tumor may represent an aggressive cancer that grew large in a short period or a lesion that has been present, but undetected, for a long time.

CONSISTENCY

The consistency of a lesion – soft, firm, hard, or cystic – is tested by securing the tumor or mass with the index finger and thumb of one hand and pressing on it with the index finger of the opposite hand. (See chapter 1, "Benign Tumors," Figure 1.5.)

Consistency varies with histologic type. On palpation, lipomas are well delineated but soft, fibroadenomas are firm, and malignant tumors are hard.

An abscess may be firm or hard in consistency. At onset, the surface is usually hard, but at the suppurative stage, the surface becomes softer, and the abscess fluctuates at the center. Tenderness and fever are usually present. The skin is red.

Fibroadenomas are solid tumors that are characteristically firm in consistency. Their consistency can be compared to the consistency of a handball (see chapter 1, "Benign Tumors," Figure 1.7) or the cartilage at the tip of the nose (see chapter 1, "Benign Tumors," Figure 1.8).

The consistency of a cyst can be compared to that of a balloon filled with water (see chapter 1, "Benign Tumors," Figure 1.50) or a blown-out cheek (Figure 1.51). Cysts containing fluid under tension may have the same firm consistency as a fibroadenoma. The difference is that a cyst "ballots" as the examiner's finger displaces the cystic fluid. The displaced fluid may also cause some discomfort during the palpation. (Fibroadenomas are painless on palpation.)

A malignant tumor has a hard consistency – "woody" or "stony" hard.

MOBILITY

Figure 6.41
Benign tumors (such as fibroadenomas) are well defined and independent of the breast tissue. For that reason, they are mobile.

On palpation, a fibroadenoma "escapes" from the examining finger (see chapter 1, "Benign Tumors," Figure 1.9).

Figure 6.42
A cyst lacks mobility. It moves only when the breast is moved. The examiner obtains a false sense

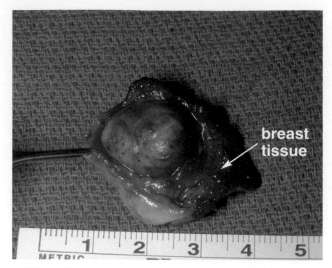

FIGURE 6.41

of mobility because the cyst moves with the breast tissue to which it is attached.

ATTACHMENT AND FIXATION

Attachment and fixation are clinical signs of locally advanced carcinoma.

Figure 6.43
To look for attachment or fixation, the examiner should stand behind the examining table and place both hands at the sides of the patient's breast. With hands in that position, he or she should try to move the breast medially and laterally.

Attachment occurs when infiltration has occurred to only one plane – for example, anteriorly to the subcutaneous tissue and skin, or posteriorly to the pectoralis major muscle. The tumor can be only partially moved.

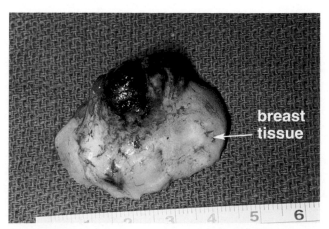

FIGURE 6.42

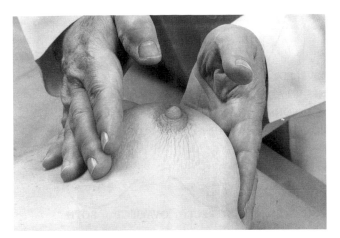

FIGURE 6.43

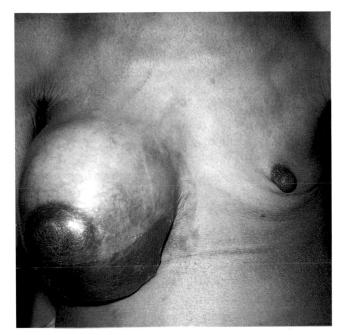

FIGURE 6.45A

Fixation occurs when infiltration has occurred to both the anterior and the posterior anatomical planes. The breast can not be moved.

The examiner can best appreciate the grade and plane (anterior or posterior) of the attachment or fixation by asking the patient to press her hands against her hips as he checks for the sign. The sign can also be appreciated if the patient elevates her arms over her head and approximates her elbows.

Figure 6.44

Figure 6.44 demonstrates attachment. The tumor has advanced locally to the subcutaneous tissue and the skin. The patient's breast could be only partially moved.

Figure 6.45A and B

Figure 6.45 (A and B) shows two different patients with locally advanced carcinoma to both planes (anterior and posterior). In each case, the patient's breast

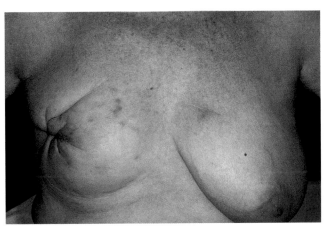

FIGURE 6.45B

cannot be moved. Today, such physical signs are seldom found, because progress in screening techniques and women's awareness of breast health have led to earlier detection of most breast cancers.

RECORDING THE DATA OBTAINED

All data obtained during a clinical visit should be recorded in a systematic fashion. With the popularity of computers today, such data can also be entered into a database and used for statistical analysis.

The history and physical examination model that follows is the one that the author uses. It is simple and practical, and it can be computerized.

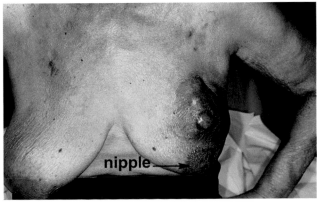

FIGURE 6.44

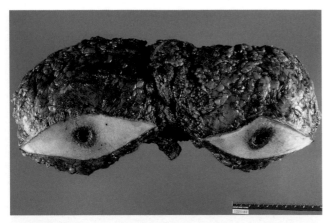

FIGURE 7.11

CLINICAL PRESENTATION

Trauma is not a cause of breast cancer. However, an injury to the breast calls for attention, leading to self-examination and the discovery of a mass.

The chief complaint of a male patient with breast carcinoma depends on the size of the tumor. Small tumors are asymptomatic. They may go undetected until they reach a large size. Large tumors may be accompanied by pain, owing to the large volume of tissue occupying a small space. The patient may seek medical assistance for the pain rather than for the mass.

Nipple discharge is rare in men. Serous or serosanguineous nipple discharge – especially if spontaneous – is likely attributable to a malignant process. (See Figure 7.12, and chapter 4, "Symptoms of the Nipple–Areola Complex," Figure 4.32.)

In women, the upper outer quadrant – the location of most of the breast tissue – is also the location of most carcinomas. In men, breast cancer is most commonly located in the nipple region – again, the place where most of the breast tissue is found. Because of the location, skin dimpling and nipple retraction are not rare (Figures 7.13 and 7.14). The skin ulceration, breast fixation, and *peau d'orange* appearance characteristic of inflammatory carcinoma are also found in men.

Axillary adenopathy is common in men with breast carcinoma. The higher incidence of axillary metastasis in men (as compared with the incidence in women) is attributable to the time that typically passes between onset of the disease and initiation of treatment in men.

Figure 7.12

In a man, spontaneous nipple discharge should raise immediate suspicion of carcinoma.

The patient in Figure 7.12 consulted because his "nipple was wet." An eczematous lesion was noted

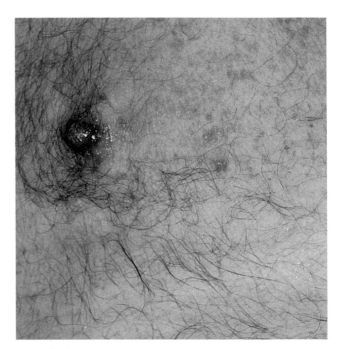

FIGURE 7.12

on the right nipple. Close observation revealed that the discharge did not come through a nipple orifice, but rather as seepage from an ulcerated area of nipple skin. A crust covered the ulcerated area. (True nipple discharge issues through a nipple orifice, is thinner, and does not form a crust.)

The clinical diagnosis of Paget's disease was confirmed from a wedge biopsy of the nipple and underlying main terminal ducts.

Figures 7.13 and 7.14

Because most breast carcinomas in men are located in the retroareolar area, nipple retraction (Figure 7.13) is a common clinical finding. This clinical sign can be observed on direct inspection or can be uncovered when the inspection is done with the patient's arms elevated or with his hands pressed to hips.

Skin and nipple involvement are more common in men than in women because of the size of the male breast and because the lesion is peripherally located. When the lesion is large and extends beyond the limits of the areola, skin dimpling can be present in addition to nipple retraction. In the patient shown in Figure 7.14, these two associated clinical findings became more evident when an inspection was done with the patient elevating his arms.

Figure 7.15

Because men seek medical attention for their breasts less frequently than women do, diagnoses of

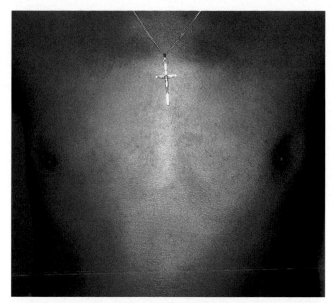

FIGURE 7.13

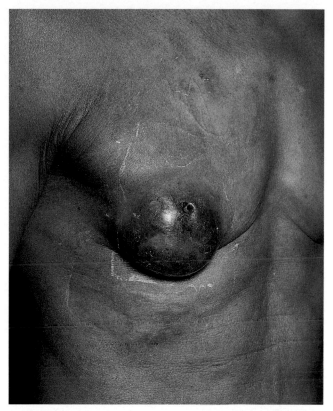

FIGURE 7.15

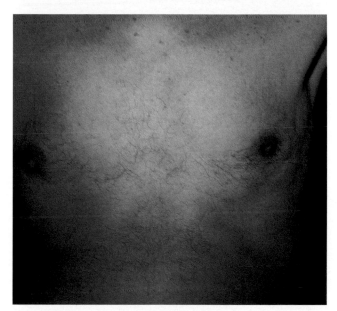

FIGURE 7.14

advanced breast cancer in men are not uncommon. In the patient shown in Figure 7.15, a carcinoma was locally advanced and fungating through the skin.

Figure 7.16

Figure 7.16 shows inflammatory carcinoma in a male patient. At the time of consultation, redness of the skin and *peau d'orange* were evident (A). The clinical diagnosis of inflammatory carcinoma was confirmed from a biopsy of the tumor and the skin. The patient received four cycles of chemotherapy to downstage the disease, with the result that the skin

edema and cellulitis subsided (B). The patient was subsequently treated with a modified radical mastectomy and additional chemotherapy.

IMAGING

The radiographic appearance of male breast cancer is similar to that of female breast cancer. The image is dense and has spiculated borders.

On ultrasonography, male breast carcinoma images as irregular and hypoechoic – no different from its female counterpart. (See chapter 8, "Role of the Radiologist.")

Figure 7.17

The mammogram in Figure 7.17 is a mediolateral oblique (MLO) projection for a 76-year-old man with breast cancer. It demonstrates a 1-cm × 1-cm tumor with slight lobulation and spiculated margins. The mass is located away from the subareolar region. On mammography, a gynecomastia images as a well-delineated density next to the subareolar region, making the differential diagnosis.

Histopathology

Because the male breast has no lobules, lobular carcinoma simply does not occur in men. The histopathologic characteristics of infiltrating ductal

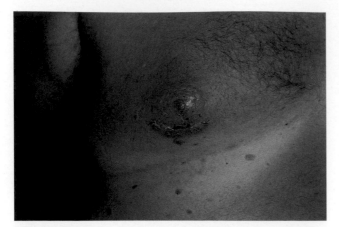

FIGURE 7.16A

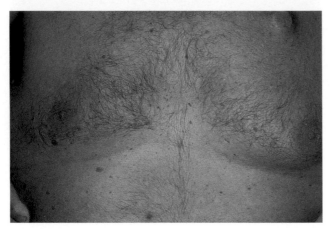

FIGURE 7.16B

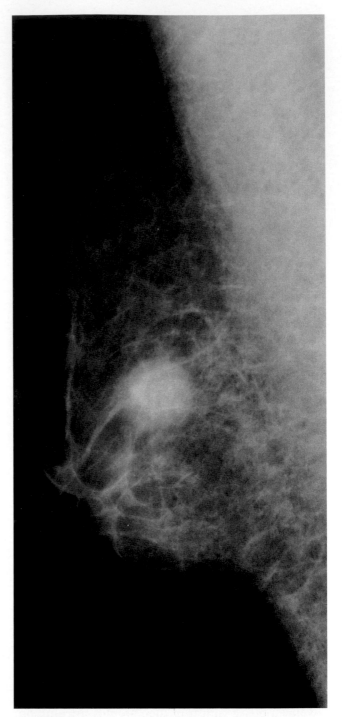

FIGURE 7.17

carcinoma in a man do not differ from those in a woman. (See chapter 9, "Role of the Pathologist.")

DIFFERENTIAL DIAGNOSIS

Differential diagnosis of a breast mass in a man is much simpler than in a woman because the male breast does not usually develop fibrocystic change and because most of the breast lesions that occur in women are rare in men.

Gynecomastia is the most common breast lesion in a man. A good history – including questions about use of medications, excessive use of alcohol, and endocrine problems – will aid in the differential diagnosis. On physical examination, gynecomastias present differently from carcinoma. The breast of a patient with gynecomastia is uniformly enlarged, well margined, and slightly tender to palpation.

TREATMENT

Breast preservation surgery – for example, lumpectomy, axillary node dissection, and radia-

tion therapy – is seldom indicated in men. The reason is that wide, clear margins are more difficult to obtain in men, owing to their smaller breast volume and, sometimes, to the proximity of the tumor to the pectoralis muscle. However, as has been the case for women, the former standard of radical mastectomy for treatment of breast cancer has been changed to modified radical mastectomy with axil-

lary node dissection. Radical mastectomy is indicated only when the cancer is attached to the pectoralis major muscle.

The surgical technique for a modified radical mastectomy in a man does not differ from that for a woman. (See chapter 12, "Surgical Treatment of Malignant Breast Lesions.").

Adjuvant radiation therapy to the chest wall may delay local recurrence, but it does not improve overall survival. Adjuvant chemotherapy is recommended for patients with large tumors and pathologic lymph nodes. Adjuvant hormonal treatment with antiestrogen is indicated for hormone-dependent tumors.

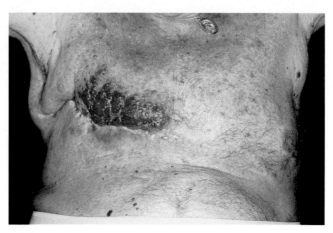

FIGURE 7.18

Figure 7.18

Locally recurrent carcinoma is more common in men because of the late stage at which the disease is typically diagnosed and because of their smaller breast volume. The 59-year-old male in Figure 7.18 was treated with a modified radical right mastectomy for a 4-cm carcinoma. The patient also received chemotherapy before and after surgery. At the time of the clinical presentation shown here, the patient was treated with radiation and additional chemotherapy.

8

Role of the Radiologist

Diagnosis

MAMMOGRAPHY
Fred Pezzulli, MD

This section is a guide to the mammography findings that a physician caring for women will most commonly encounter. It familiarizes clinicians with the types of mammograms that they may be reviewing during an office consultation.

Types of Mammography

Mammography is either screening or diagnostic.

SCREENING MAMMOGRAPHY

Asymptomatic women undergo screening mammography with the goal of detecting a carcinoma early. The American College of Radiology and the U.S. National Cancer Institute recommend that women have a baseline mammogram at age 35–40, and annual mammograms thereafter. Family history and other risk factors (early menarche, nulliparity, and late parity) are used to modify the recommendation. For example, if a woman's mother had breast carcinoma at age 39, the recommendation is that screening begin five years earlier – that is, no later than age 34.

DIAGNOSTIC MAMMOGRAPHY

Diagnostic mammography evaluates a specific clinical or mammographic abnormality. For example, a clinically palpable mass should be evaluated using routine views, plus additional views of the area of question (spot-magnification views, for instance). If the mammograms fail to reveal an abnormality, then the area should be evaluated using ultrasonography. An abnormality detected during routine screening mammography should be further evaluated by additional views. Those views could include spot compressions, rotation views, and exaggerated-angle views, among others. Ultrasonography should be used to evaluate any masses or areas of asymmetric density.

Mammographic Analysis

The first step in analyzing a mammogram is to determine if the image is technically adequate.

Mammograms should be viewed in a predetermined sequence. The mediolateral oblique (MLO) projection (Figure 8.1 [A and B]) and cranial-caudal (CC) projection (Figure 8.2 [A and B]) of the right and the left breast are placed back-to-back so that the two sides can be compared. When unilateral mammograms are obtained, additional views, if any, should be placed in proximity to the standard views. (In addition to the standard MLO and CC projections, the clinical presentation may require exaggerated CC views (Figure 8.3 [A and B]), cleavage views (Figure 8.4 [A and B]), and spot-compression views (Figure 8.5 [A and B]).)

The positioning of the exposures should be such that the glandular and fatty elements of the breast and any faint microcalcifications or subtle densities are well visualized. If the positioning or the exposures are suboptimal, a repeat examination should be scheduled when clinically feasible. Necessary rescheduling often causes concern to the patient, but an explanation of the necessity of adequate positioning and exposure for accurate diagnosis is generally well accepted.

Normal mammograms range from those that are almost entirely fat-replaced to those that are completely dense. The completely dense mammogram poses a special problem, in that masses and faint calcifications are often obscured. Special care must be exercised in evaluating a dense mammogram. It is well known that a certain percentage of dense mammograms will contain malignancies that cannot be seen. Consequently, a report of "normal mammo-

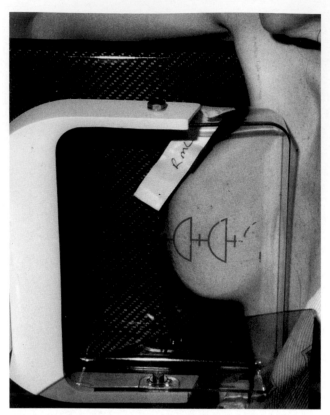

FIGURE 8.1A

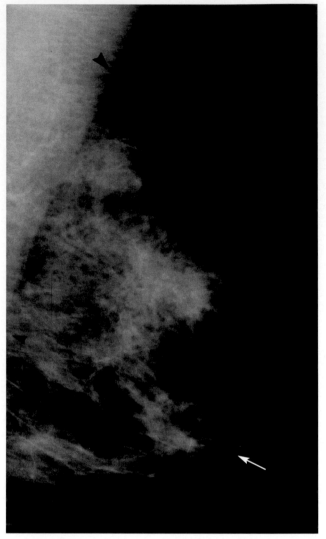

FIGURE 8.1B

gram" must be tempered with that knowledge. Ultra-sonography should be used liberally if a palpable mass or thickening has been found.

Figure 8.1A and 8.1B

In the mediolateral oblique (MLO) projection, the pectoral muscle (large arrow) should be well visualized and symmetrical. The inferior extent of the muscle should be seen to the mid-plane of the mammogram at least, and the nipple should be in profile and parallel (small arrows). The inframammary fold should be well visualized to ensure that the post-inferior portion of the breast is included.

Figure 8.2A and 8.2B

In the cranial-caudal (CC) projection, the nipple should be seen in profile. Ideally, a portion of the pectoral muscle should be seen along the posterior margin of the film (arrows).

Figure 8.3A and 8.3B

In the exaggerated cranial-caudal (CC) projection, the shoulder is brought forward and rotated (A) to better visualize the upper outer quadrant (UOQ) of the breast and the tail of Spence. High in the UOQ of left breast, the mammogram images a spiculated le-

sion [(B), arrow] that was partly obscured on the regular CC view.

Figure 8.4A and 8.4B

In a cleavage view, the inner quadrants of both breasts are simultaneously imaged. This additional view is taken for breast lesions located in the middle quadrants and close to the sternum.

Figure 8.5A and 8.5B

The spot-compression view is used to better evaluate densities that may represent superimposed glandular tissue rather than a tumor (also see Figure 8.22), or to better image calcifications.

Abnormal Mammographic Findings

The most common mammographic findings are calcifications and soft-tissue densities. Calcifications are

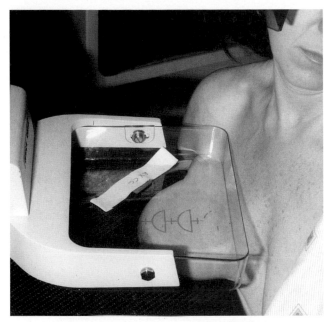

FIGURE 8.2A

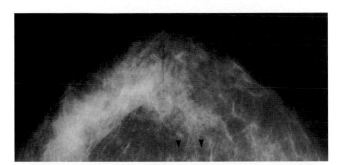

FIGURE 8.2B

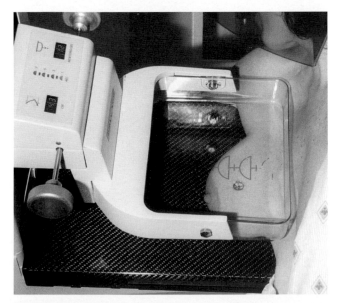

FIGURE 8.3A

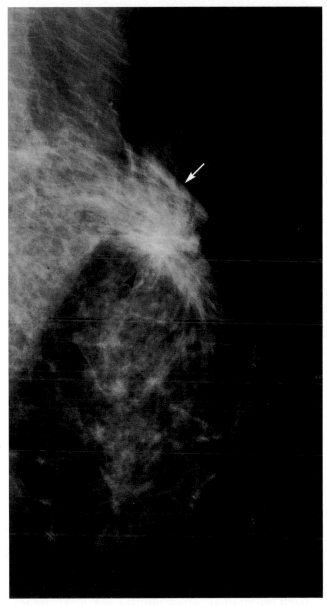

FIGURE 8.3B

classified as typically benign, probably benign, suspicious (indeterminate), or typically malignant. The determination is based on an evaluation of morphology and distribution. Abnormal soft-tissue densities include nodules, masses, asymmetric densities, and architectural distortion.

Only the most common mammographic findings in each category are discussed here. Several types were included in the clinical chapters, and so, to avoid repetition, readers are referred to those chapters.

TYPICALLY BENIGN CALCIFICATIONS

The "typically benign" calcification types most commonly imaged on mammograms are vascular

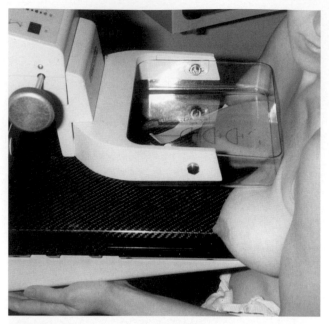

FIGURE 8.4A

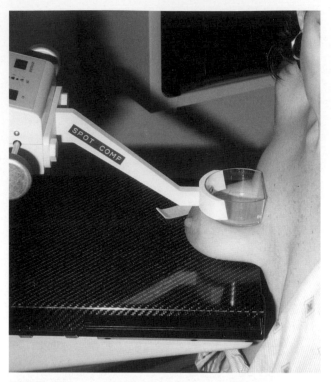

FIGURE 8.5A

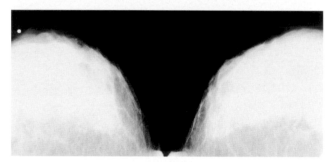

FIGURE 8.4B

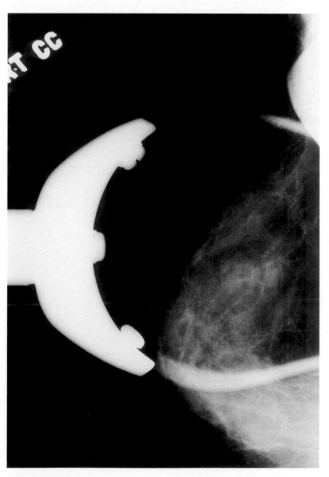

FIGURE 8.5B

calcifications, sebaceous gland calcifications, plasma cell mastitis calcifications, eggshell calcifications, milk of calcium calcifications, sutural calcifications, coarse dystrophic calcifications, and lobular calcifications.

Most **vascular calcifications** have a typical appearance that resembles vascular calcifications elsewhere in the body (Figure 8.6). Occasionally, irregular vascular calcifications can be mistaken for the branching intraductal calcifications seen in ductal carcinoma in situ [(DCIS), see Figure 8.19]. In those cases, biopsy is the only definitive means of diagnosis.

Sebaceous gland calcifications are ring-like calcifications in the skin (Figures 8.7 and 8.8). They generally appear in multiples. Tangential views can be used to locate them to the skin.

Milk of calcium calcifications frequently form within dilated lobules during adenosis. They can be semisolid, and they can vary in appearance in differ-

ent projections (smudgy on the CC view and a sharply marginated teacup shape on a 90-degree lateral projection.

Sutural calcifications are the result of granuloma and fat necrosis along the direction of a suture line (Figure 8.9).

Coarse dystrophic ("popcorn") calcifications are frequently seen in involuting fibroadenomas (see Figure 8.12 and Figures 1.15 and 1.16 in Chapter 1, "Reasons for Breast Consultations").

Benign **lobular calcifications** are smoothly marginated and rounded. They may be single, loosely grouped, or widely scattered.

Skin calcifications are generally rounded and smoothly marginated. They may be mistaken for parenchymal calcifications unless special views are taken tangential to the skin (see Figure 8.13).

Figure 8.6

Vascular calcifications like those in Figure 8.6 are more common in patients of advanced age. They are characterized by their serpentine shape, the calcium having been deposited along the wall of the blood vessel. Vascular calcifications in the breast are no different from those seen in other parts of the body.

Figure 8.7

A 49-year-old patient had had a lumpectomy for ductal carcinoma in situ (DCIS). Several years later, a postoperative follow-up mammogram (Figure 8.7) imaged multiple smoothly marginated, lucid-centered calcifications within the skin of the axilla. They were typical of sebaceous gland calcifications. Tangential views confirmed that the calcifications were located in the skin and not in the tail of Spence.

Figure 8.8

A patient 35 years of age consulted because of a mammography finding of breast calcifications. Her mother had had breast carcinoma. On examination,

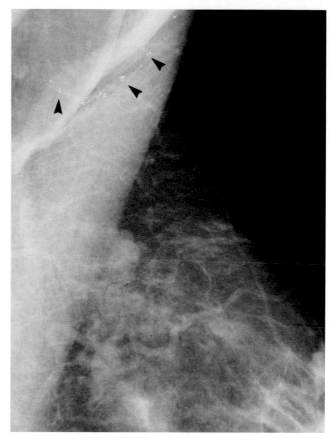

FIGURE 8.7

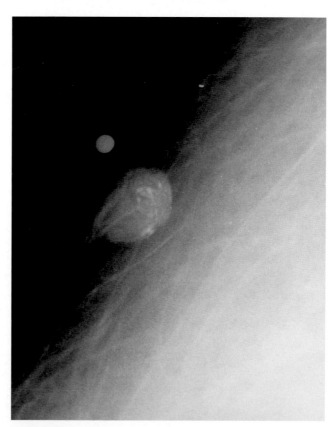

FIGURE 8.8

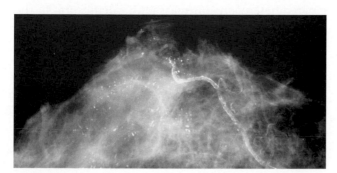

FIGURE 8.6

a nodule was found in an upper quadrant of her right breast, corresponding to the area where the calcifications had been imaged. The nodule measured approximately 1 cm in diameter and was stone-hard to palpation.

Histopathology was consistent with a calcified epithelioma of the sebaceous gland (known as a calcifying epithelioma of Malherbe). Because of differentiation toward hair structures, this entity is also known as pilomatricoma.

Pilomatricomas are tumors that can occur anywhere in the body, but that are more common in the face and upper extremities. The smoothly marginated nodule with coarse calcifications resembles a calcified fibroadenoma or a carcinoma (see Fitzpatrick 1999 in "Suggested Readings.")

Figure 8.9

A patient was treated with lumpectomy, axillary dissection, and radiation therapy for a breast carcinoma. Her follow-up mediolateral oblique (MLO) projection mammogram (Figure 8.9) images irregular, rounded, and curved calcifications following the direction of a suture line. The suture material calcified as the result of the surrounding granuloma and fat necrosis. A history of previous surgery and the typical linear arrangement are characteristic of this type of calcification.

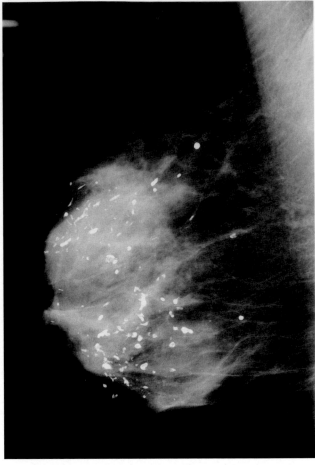

FIGURE 8.10

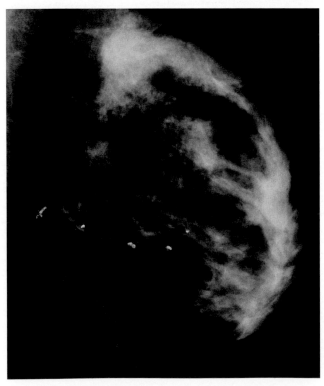

FIGURE 8.9

Figure 8.10

Rod-shaped calcifications are typically seen in breast secretory disease such as chronic duct ectasia. They differ from the linear calcifications seen in ductal carcinoma in situ (DCIS) because they are larger in size (> 0.5 cm) and they do not branch.

Figure 8.11

A patient consulted because of a mass found on self-examination. The cranial-caudal (CC) projection of the breast (Figure 8.11) demonstrated a well-marginated heterogeneous mass with calcification in the wall and a lucent center characteristic of fat necrosis ("oil cyst" with calcification) (arrow). Further history revealed that the patient had sustained a car accident and developed ecchymosis in the skin of the breast where the seat belt had restrained her. (See chapter 5, "Skin Symptoms," Figure 5.3.)

Figure 8.12

The mediolateral oblique (MLO) projection mammogram in Figure 8.12 imaged coarse calcifica-

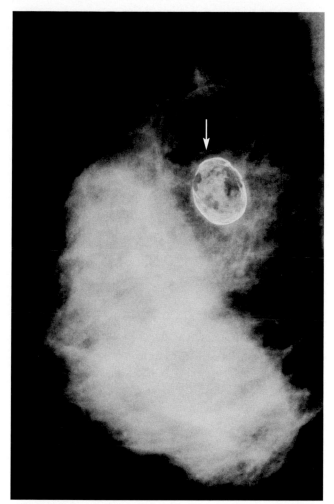

FIGURE 8.11

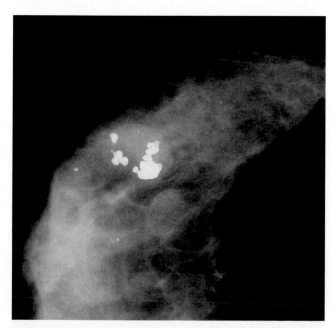

FIGURE 8.12

tions within a soft-tissue mass. This "popcorn" type of dystrophic calcification is characteristic of an involuting fibroadenoma.

Figure 8.13

The multiple ring-like calcifications in this mammogram appeared to follow a ductal pattern [Figure 8.13(A) (arrow)]. Because of the patient's family history of breast cancer, surgery was recommended. During the attempted localization, using tangential views, the calcifications were found to be within the skin [Figure 8.13(B)]. Calcifications that cannot be localized in two projections should raise a suspicion of dermal calcifications.

PROBABLY BENIGN CALCIFICATIONS

The probably benign group of calcifications may require histopathology diagnosis despite a very low probability of malignancy (Figure 8.14).

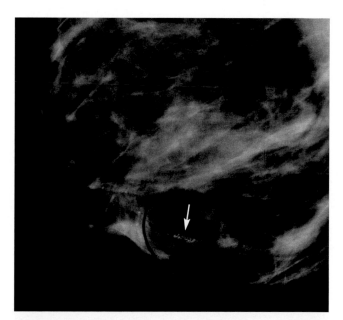

FIGURE 8.13A

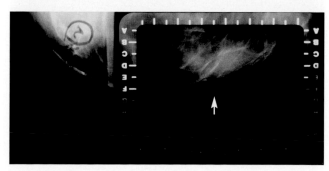

FIGURE 8.13B

SUSPICIOUS CALCIFICATIONS

Suspicious calcifications image as

- smoothly marginated calcifications in clusters of five or more within a 1-cm area (more commonly found in non-comedo DCIS – for example, cribriform or micropapillary).
- slightly irregular, loosely grouped calcifications.
- pleomorphic but non-branching calcifications.

TYPICALLY MALIGNANT CALCIFICATIONS

Calcifications are highly suggestive of malignancy when they image as

- heterogeneous and pleomorphic.
- linear and branching irregular intraductal calcifications (more common in DCIS with significant necrosis – for example, comedo DCIS).

Figure 8.14
The smoothly marginated calcifications of sclerosing adenosis are typically scattered throughout

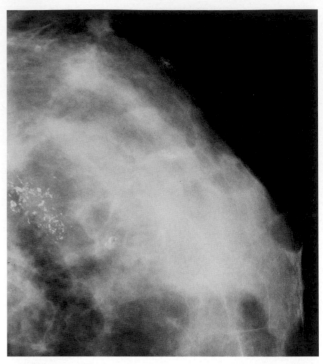

FIGURE 8.15

the breast, but they may also be loosely clustered. Calcifications of sclerosing adenosis are commonly bilateral.

Figure 8.15
A cranial-caudal (CC) projection mammogram with magnification images two groups of pleomorphic calcifications in the lateral aspect of the breast.

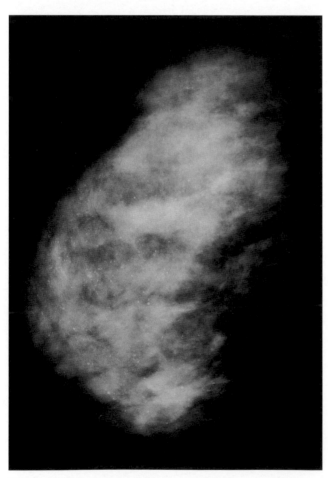

FIGURE 8.14

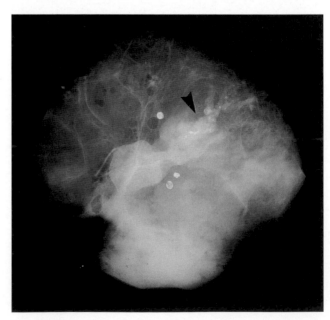

FIGURE 8.16

The larger group has a branching tendency, consistent with a malignancy.

Figure 8.16

A specimen radiograph demonstrates a lobulated and spiculated mass (malignant tumor) with associated pleomorphic microcalcifications (arrow). Several associated benign microcalcifications are also seen.

Figures 8.17 and 8.18

A mediolateral (ML) projection mammogram for a 54-year-old patient images a cluster of smooth microcalcifications in the upper medial quadrant and several other areas of typical lobular calcifications (Figure 8.17). Because the first cluster was of an indeterminate category, excision of an adjacent group of calcifications was also recommended. Two localizations were required (Figure 8.18). The first cluster represented an infiltrating ductal carcinoma; the second represented adenosis.

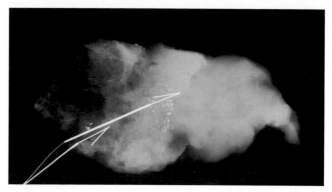

FIGURE 8.18

Figure 8.19

A mediolateral (ML) projection mammogram demonstrates the typical extensive branching of malignant calcifications. The axilla shows enlarged, homogeneously dense lymph nodes (arrows) consistent with metastasis.

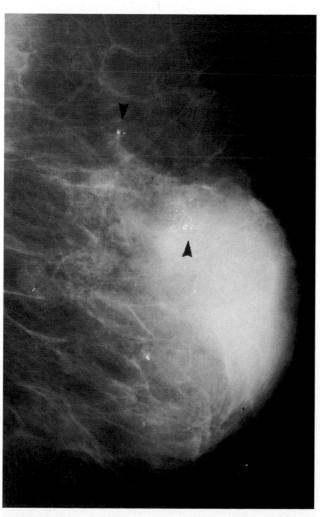

FIGURE 8.17

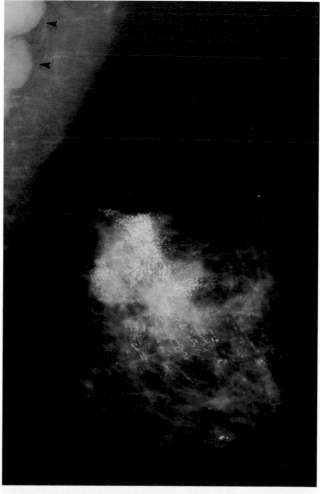

FIGURE 8.19

Figure 8.20
A magnification-view mammogram centers on the typical extensive branching of malignant calcifications in a patient with ductal and infiltrating ductal carcinoma.

SOFT-TISSUE DENSITIES
Benign Masses
The benign masses most commonly seen in practice are

- Intramammary nodes
- Cysts
- Lipomas
- Galactoceles
- Hamartomas
- Skin moles
- Keloids

Benign **intramammary and axillary nodes** are generally found in the outer portion of the breast. They have a smoothly marginated reniform appearance with a notch at the hilum of the node. On ultrasonography, a smooth nodule with an echogenic center is characteristic.

Figure 8.21
In a mediolateral oblique (MLO) projection mammogram, the kidney-shaped nodule with a lu-

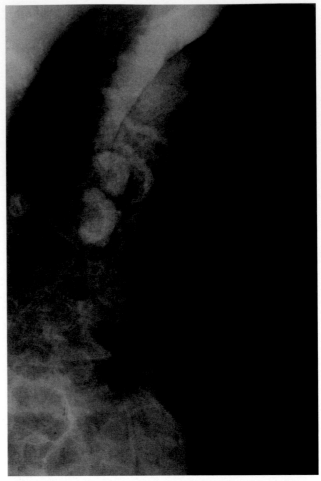

FIGURE 8.21

cent hilum (arrow) is consistent with a normal axillary lymph node. Lymph nodes with metastatic disease are homogeneously dense (see Figure 8.19).

Benign **cysts** are smoothly marginated nodules that occasionally contain a thin rim of calcifications on the cyst wall. The cyst may be partly obscured by dense glandular tissue and only partly visualized. Ultrasound is characteristic, demonstrating an anechoic center with through transmission of the sound beam (see chapter 1, "Benign Tumors," Figures 1.55 through 1.58.)

Lipomas present as areas of well-marginated lucency with a thin capsule. Calcification of the capsule may occur.

Galactoceles are milk-containing cysts that occur during or immediately after lactation. They contain a mixture of retained milk and fat. On mammography, they are smoothly marginated and heterogeneous.

Hamartomas ("fibroadenolipomas") are masses containing glandular, mesenchymal, and fatty tissue. Characteristically, they are well margined, with a

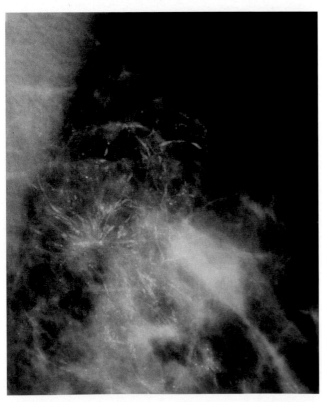

FIGURE 8.20

thin capsule that separates the lesion from the adjacent breast tissue. On ultrasonography, hamartomas present with a heterogeneous internal echo pattern reflecting the various fibrous, glandular, and fatty elements contained within (see chapter 1, "Benign Tumors," Figure 1.22).

Probably Benign Masses

The probably benign masses most commonly imaged in daily practice are

- Asymmetry
- Fibroadenomas (and giant fibroadenomas)
- Phyllodes tumors
- Radial scars
- Hemangiomas
- Papillomas
- Hematomas
- Granular cell tumors
- Abscesses
- Seromas

Benign **asymmetry** usually reflects asymmetric distribution of glandular tissue. The density is non-palpable and compressible on spot-compression films. It often has the heterogeneous appearance of normal glandular tissue. The finding should be corroborated using ultrasonography.

Fibroadenomas are soft-tissue masses that may calcify when they undergo involution.

Non-calcified fibroadenomas present as soft-tissue nodules that may be oval-shaped or lobulated (see chapter 1, "Benign Tumors," Figures 1.3 and 1.6). A definitive diagnosis cannot be made using mammography. On ultrasonography, typical fibroadenomas are oval shaped and sharply marginated with a thin, echogenic capsule. They demonstrate homogenous internal echoes (see chapter 1, "Benign Tumors," Figure 1.14). If a lesion meets these three criteria, it may be followed sonographically or excised depending on the level of the patient's anxiety over "having a lump on the breast."

Calcified fibroadenomas may present with typically large, coarse, dystrophic calcifications or with more indeterminate calcifications. In the latter case, a biopsy is recommended, because the morphology of the calcifications should be the determining factor.

A fibroadenoma variant is the giant fibroadenoma, which typically presents in young patients. Its mammographic features are similar to those of fibroadenoma. Because the need for cosmesis results in the excision of giant fibroadenomas sooner than is the case with fibroadenomas, calcifications in giant fibroadenomas are seldom seen.

Phyllodes tumors can be benign or malignant. Conventionally, these tumors have been called "cystosarcoma phyllodes." More recently, the terms benign and malignant phyllodes tumor are more commonly used. Phyllodes tumors are fibroadenoma variants, in which epithelial and mesenchymal elements are both present.

From an imaging perspective, distinguishing between malignant and benign phyllodes tumors, and between phyllodes tumors and fibroadenomas is often difficult. In most cases, the tumors are smoothly marginated lobular masses. The larger the tumor, the higher the likelihood of its being malignant. On ultrasonography, a benign phyllodes tumor may exhibit the typical characteristics of a benign fibroadenoma. In other cases, the internal architecture may show cystic spaces and an inhomogeneous echo texture. A definitive diagnosis requires tissue sampling, which can be done by stereotactic Mammotome biopsy or ultrasound-guided core biopsy.

Radial scars consist of entrapped breast tissue presenting as a spiculated architectural distortion mimicking scirrhous carcinoma. The lesions frequently have a central lucent core with elongated radiating spicules. Their appearance varies in different projections. Calcifications are commonly present. Ultrasound generally shows an irregular-shaped hypoechoic mass.

Because tubular carcinoma is associated with radial scars in about 15%–20% of cases, the lesion is routinely treated using surgical excision. The lesion is not ideally suited for core biopsy, because the associated carcinoma is often found at a distance from the central core of the radial scar, and a definitive diagnosis can rarely be made from the biopsy. Most radial scars are microscopic, ranging between 0.3 cm and 0.6 cm in diameter. They are often found incidentally at biopsy for other lesions. (See Chapter 9, "The Role of the Pathologist," Figures 9.39, 9.40 and 9.41.)

Hemangiomas occur in the breast just as in other parts of the body. They generally present as dense masses (often containing calcified phlebolith). They may be bilateral. On ultrasonography, they have a heterogeneous internal architecture reflecting the varying tissue components. When calcifications are present, marked posterior shadowing is seen (see chapter 5, "Skin Symptoms," Figure 5.6).

Papillomas are intraductal lesions. They may be centrally located in the subareolar region or more peripherally located (see chapter 4, "Symptoms of the Nipple–Areola complex," Figure 4.37). Central intraductal papillomas are rarely imaged on a mammogram. Peripheral lesions present as single or multiple nodular densities. Dystrophic calcifications may occur

within papillomas. On ultrasonography, they present as lobulated hypoechoic lesions (see Figure 8.41).

Granular cell tumors are not specific tumors of the breast. They are almost invariably benign, but their spiculated margin mimics a carcinoma on radiographs (see chapter 2, "Malignant Tumors," Figures 2.8, 2.11, and 2.12).

Figure 8.22

Asymmetry can be technical, or it can be attributed to an increased amount of breast tissue in part of the breast. A spot-compression magnification view (see Figure 8.5) displaces the breast parenchyma and improves the imaging of fine details.

Figure 8.22 is a cranial–caudal (CC) view mammogram that shows an asymmetry attributable to the presence of a spiculated mass in the posterior and central segment of the left breast.

Figure 8.23

Fibroadenomas are smooth and have a sharply defined margin. When the epithelial elements of the tumor are encircled and compressed by fibrous tissue, a fibroadenoma can also image as a lobulated mass (see chapter 1, "Benign Tumors," Figures 1.3, 1.4, and 1.6).

Figure 8.24

Figure 8.24 shows the mammogram of a patient whose pre-localization film demonstrated a spiculated mass in the upper portion of the breast. That mass raised a high suspicion of malignancy. On localization, the lesion lacked a central mass. It was an area of architectural distortion with elastic tissue at its center. The center had lucent zones. (See chapter 9, "Role of the Pathologist," Figures 9.39–9.41.)

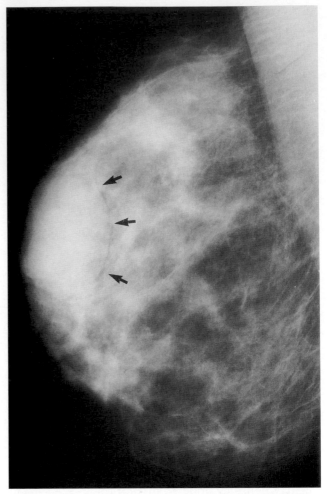

FIGURE 8.23

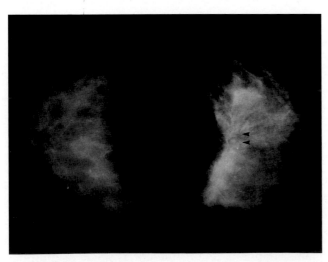

FIGURE 8.22

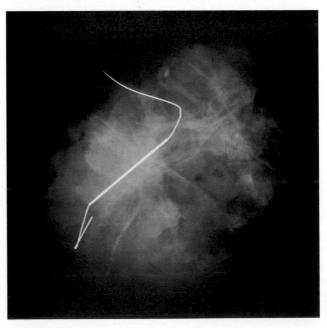

FIGURE 8.24

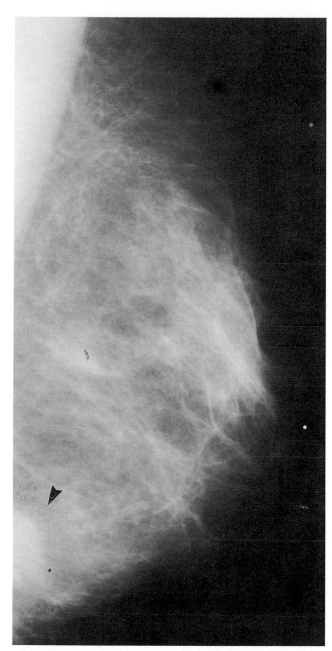

FIGURE 8.25

Figure 8.25
A mediolateral oblique (MLO) projection mammogram images a granular cell tumor as a well-marginated mass with spiculation resembling a carcinoma (arrow).

SOFT-TISSUE DENSITIES SUSPICIOUS OR HIGHLY SUGGESTIVE OF MALIGNANCY

Any lesion – with or without associated calcification – that cannot be considered benign or probably benign should be considered for biopsy. Morphologically, these lesions cover a broad range of categories. (It is important to note that a mass and its associated calcifications should be analyzed separately.)

- Lobulated nodules or masses
  The more lobulations within a nodule or mass, the more suspicious the lesion. If a sonographically solid nodule or mass shows more than three lobulations (and especially if they are microlobulations), a biopsy should be done.
- Spiculated densities
  Many spiculated densities – such as radial scars and areas of fat necrosis – are benign. If a benign or probably benign cause cannot be established by other means, a biopsy should be done. Spiculated carcinomas can range from a few millimeters to several centimeters in size. If no central mass is associated with the spiculation, a core biopsy may not be diagnostic, and excisional biopsy recommended.
- New, enlarging densities
  Any new density should be viewed with suspicion, and a biopsy should be considered. The same applies to existing densities that enlarge over time.

Figure 8.26
The cranial–caudal (CC) projection mammogram in Figure 8.26 demonstrates an irregular 3-cm × 1-cm mass with spiculated margins. No associated calcifications are seen. Skin retraction is noted with this carcinoma.

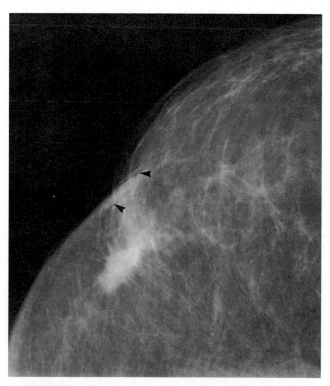

FIGURE 8.26

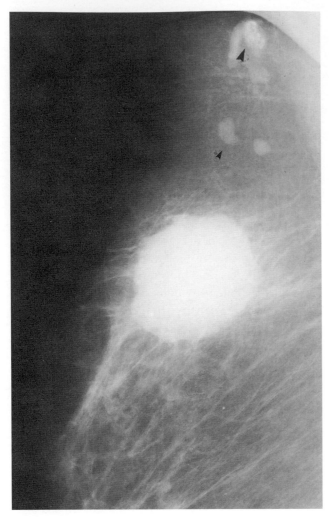

FIGURE 8.27

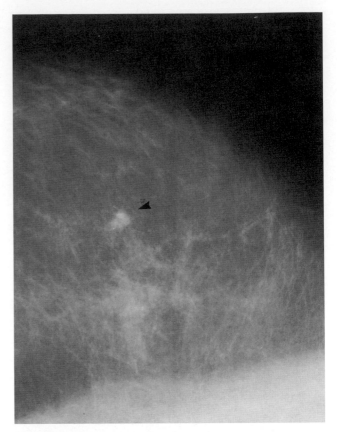

FIGURE 8.28A

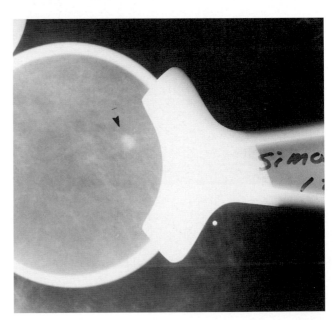

FIGURE 8.28B

Figure 8.27

The mammogram in Figure 8.27 images an irregular rounded mass measuring 3.4 cm × 4 cm. The border is slightly lobulated and contains thin, irregular spicules extending toward the parenchyma, the largest toward the nipple. Rounded calcifications are noted in the anterior margin. The axillary (large arrow) and intramammary nodes (small arrow) are also imaged. The axillary node shows dystrophic calcifications. The intramammary and axillary nodes were both metastatic.

Figure 8.28A and 8.28B

An oblique projection mammogram of the left breast demonstrates a small nodule with faintly spiculated margins (A). A spot-compression view (B) indicates that the nodule is not compressible and better visualizes the spiculated margins. The lesion was an infiltrating carcinoma.

Figure 8.29

Figure 8.29 is a mammographic view of a retroareolar carcinoma with nipple retraction (arrow). The 2-cm, lobulated, spiculated mass was

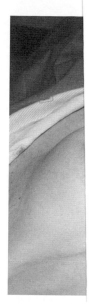

FIGURE 8.32

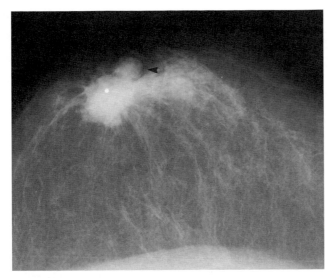

FIGURE 8.29

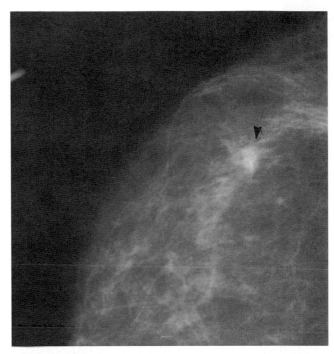

FIGURE 8.30A

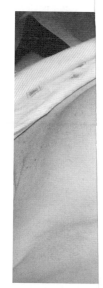

FIGURE 8.33

Figure 8.34

The norm
breast ultrason
tissues (B), fibr
muscles (D) an

SKIN

Skin is nor
transducer as a
2 mm in thick
be seen in con
(as in venous o
ure), after loca
breast cancer.

located in the inferior retroareolar portion of the breast.

Figure 8.30

A cranial–caudal (CC) projection mammogram demonstrates a 4-mm × 6-mm spiculated nodule in the outer portion of the breast (A). The mammogram from one year earlier (B) showed faint areas of increased density that were non-diagnostic for malignancy. This developing density was a manifestation of an infiltrating carcinoma.

Classification System for Mammography Findings

The American College of Radiology has created a classification system called BIRADS (Breast Imaging Reporting and Data System) for mammography findings. The intent of the system is to standardize mammography reports and to make recommendations for further management. The system classifies mammography findings into one of six categories:

- Category 0 (zero): Incomplete assessment. Additional work-up required.
- Category I: Negative (N). Routine follow-up.
- Category II: Benign (B). Routine follow-up.
- Category III: Probably benign (P). Short-interval follow-up.
- Category IV: Suspicious anomaly (S). Biopsy recommended.
- Category V: Highly suggestive of malignancy (M). Biopsy mandatory.

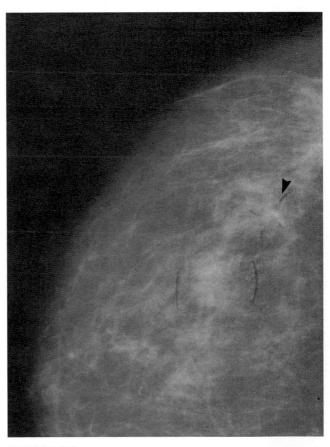

FIGURE 8.30B

Left column (partial / cut off)

BREA

EVAN

When f
primaril
lesions
mogran
sonogra
the cha
sion of
patholo
based o
be furth
probabil
be follov
uation v

Typi
include
mammo
ties. Cur
phy has
procedu
young p
cally der
to evalu
resonanc
examina

**Overvie
Examir**

Breast ul
Unlike m
quire the
ionizing

The
patient ii
the ipsil
That pos
chest wal

A sm
coupling
sound tr
frequency

Vario
breast. Th
in the tra
moved ir
the nippl

Wher
tained in
anti-radia

Middle column

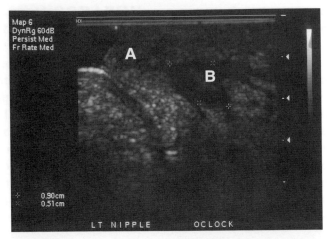

FIGURE 8.35

lump. The nipple (A) and a small mass (B) behind the nipple can be seen in the sonogram.

Figure 8.36

Ultrasonography can frequently detect the lymph nodes in the axillary portion of the breast, as well as those within the breast (intramammary lymph nodes). Figure 8.36 shows the typical sonographic appearance of an intramammary lymph node. Lymph nodes throughout the body demonstrate a hypoechoic periphery (A) (the lymphatic tissue) and central echogenic hilum (the normal fatty hilum [B]).

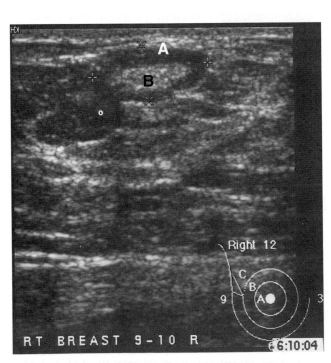

FIGURE 8.36

Right column

If the hilum has been replaced with tissue that is more hypoechoic, the structure can be difficult to identify as a node. But if such a configuration is seen, the possibility of neoplastic involvement should be raised.

Abnormalities Seen with Breast Ultrasonography

Once the normal structures are familiar to the examiner, abnormalities within those normal structures can be identified.

SIMPLE CYST

Simple cysts are usually easy to document with ultrasonography. The ultrasound criteria for this lesion are

- an anechoic internal matrix (completely black on the sonogram).
- enhanced through transmission (tissues directly behind the cyst are brighter than the surrounding tissue because the ultrasound beam is not attenuated as it passes through the fluid of a cyst in the same manner as it is attenuated by the tissue around the cyst).
- a sharply defined thin wall.

Simple cysts usually require no further evaluation unless the patient is symptomatic or requires relief from the psychological stress of having "something" in her breast. In those instances, a fine-needle aspiration can be performed.

Figure 8.37

Figure 8.37 shows the sonographic appearance of a simple cyst. The internal matrix is completely ane-

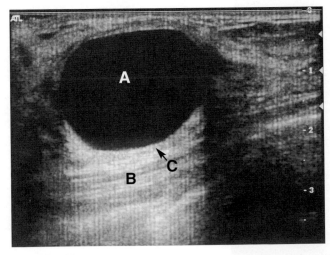

FIGURE 8.37

choic (A), through transmission is enhanced (B), and a thin, barely perceptible wall is present (C).

COMPLEX CYSTS

Certain cystic lesions do not meet the criteria of a simple cyst. These include cysts that contain septa or low-level echoes (Figures 8.38 through 8.40).

If such a lesion demonstrates enhanced through transmission and a sharply defined, thin wall, it can frequently be classified as a complex cyst. However, that appearance may be difficult to distinguish from a very hypoechoic solid lesion. In those instances, aspiration can be attempted. Then, if no material is aspirated, a biopsy may be performed. Alternatively, if differentiation between a complex cyst and a probably benign, hypoechoic solid lesion is impossible, the patient can be recalled for a short-interval follow-up at six months.

Of more concern are complex cystic lesions that contain mural nodules. These may be intraductal papillomas, with the cystic part of the lesion being a dilated duct. However, the same appearance may also be seen with the relatively uncommon cystic papillary carcinoma. Therefore, when a cyst with one or more mural nodules is encountered, a biopsy should be recommended.

Figures 8.38, 8.39, and 8.40

Figures 8.38–8.40 are sonograms of complex cysts, including a cyst with septation (Figure 8.38 [arrow]), a cyst with septa and low-level echoes (Figure 8.39 [arrow]), and a cyst filled with low-level echoes (A) (Figure 8.40).

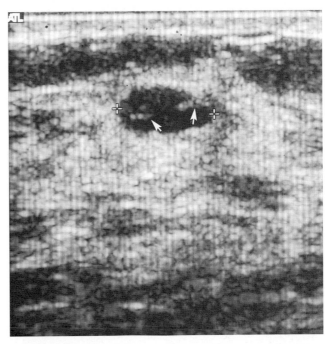

FIGURE 8.39

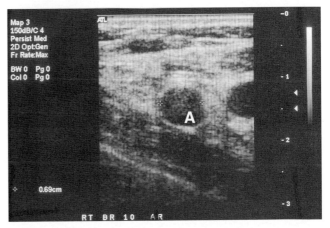

FIGURE 8.40

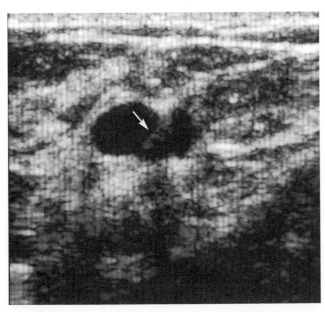

FIGURE 8.38

Figure 8.41

The tubular cystic structure with multiple mural nodules (A) in Figure 8.41 represents a dilated duct with intraductal papillomas (arrows).

PROBABLY BENIGN SOLID NODULES

Solid breast nodules imaged using ultrasonography may be subdivided into those that are likely benign and those that are indeterminate or suspicious. The sonographic features of a probably benign solid nodule are

- smooth borders (or, at most, three gentle lobulations).

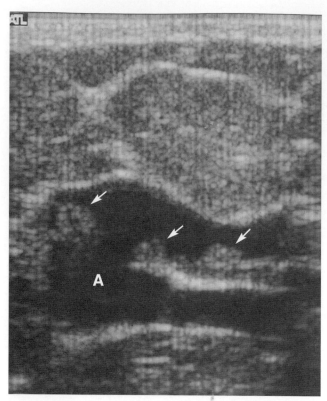

FIGURE 8.41

more apparent upon remembering that the normal tissue planes within the breast run parallel to chest wall. Benign tumors tend to grow *along* the normal tissue planes; malignant lesions grow *through* them.

An examiner can also detect the coarse "popcorn" type of calcification frequently seen in fibroadenomas on ultrasound examination. These calcifications appear as very bright echogenic foci with distal acoustic shadowing (Figure 8.43).

The distal acoustic shadowing is the result of the ultrasound beam being unable to penetrate beyond the calcification. No information distal to it is recorded on the sonogram; it appears completely black.

Other pathologic conditions can also have the appearance of a benign nodule on a sonogram. These include papillomas, areas of hyalinized fibrosis, fibrocystic disease, and adenosis, among others.

Figure 8.42

Figure 8.42 demonstrates the sonographic appearance of a fibroadenoma: ovoid, smooth-bordered solid nodule (A), with its long axis parallel to the chest wall and a thin, echogenic capsule on its periphery.

Figure 8.43

Figure 8.43 shows a fibroadenoma with coarse calcification (A) and posterior shadowing (B).

INDETERMINATE AND SUSPICIOUS NODULES

Any nodule that fails to meet all of the criteria for a probably benign nodule is classified as either indeterminate or suspicious. It should therefore be biopsied.

The appearance of such lesions is variable. Suspicious nodules can demonstrate both enhanced through transmission and distal shadowing, limiting

- a thin echogenic capsule around the entire periphery of the nodule.
- a long axis that is parallel to the chest wall [that is to say that the lesion cannot be "taller than it is wide" (Figure 8.42)].

If a lesion meets all of the criteria of a probably benign nodule, the patient can be offered the option of a biopsy or of follow-up studies every six months over a two- to three-year period. If follow-up is chosen, and the nodule remains stable during that time, the lesion can generally be considered benign, with no further work-up required. If, however, during the course of the follow-up, the lesion changes in size or appearance, a biopsy should be recommended. If biopsy is chosen or required, the physician may discuss with the patient possible alternatives (percutaneous imaging-guided biopsy or surgical biopsy).

The most commonly encountered benign solid breast nodule is the fibroadenoma.

Given the usual gross anatomic and mammographic appearances of benign solid breast lesions such as fibroadenomas, the first two of the probably benign criteria are almost intuitive. That is to say that these lesions usually have smooth borders on gross anatomic inspection and mammography alike, and they are well encapsulated. The logic for the third criterion becomes

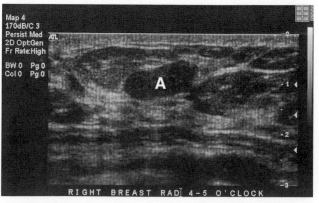

FIGURE 8.42

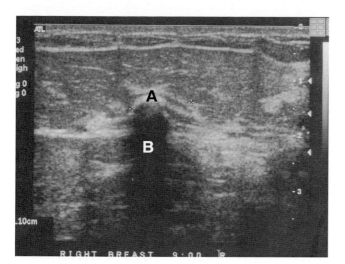

FIGURE 8.43

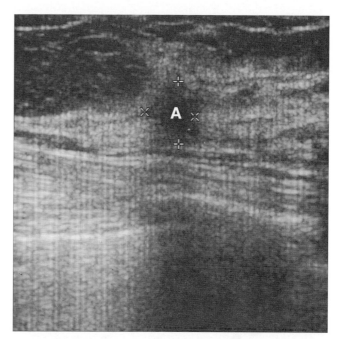

FIGURE 8.44

the value of those features. However, the most typical appearance for a suspicious nodule is a poorly defined hypoechoic mass, taller than it is wide, with irregular or microlobulated margins (Figures 8.44, 8.45, and 8.46). When such a lesion is seen, malignancy should be highly suspected.

The most common malignancy seen is infiltrating ductal carcinoma. Other malignancies such as invasive lobular cancer, metastatic disease, and lymphoma (Figure 8.46) can also be imaged. However, the latter two entities may present a more well-defined nodule than is seen with typical primary breast carcinoma.

Benign lesions can demonstrate features of an indeterminate nodule. Some fibroadenomas do not meet all of the criteria of a probably benign nodule. The same can be true of a variety of other lesions such as focal fibrosis, fibrocystic disease, fat necrosis, and adenosis.

Figures 8.44, 8.45, and 8.46

Figures 8.44, 8.45, and 8.46 show sonograms of suspicious nodules. The sonogram of an infiltrating ductal carcinoma (Figure 8.44 [A]) shows a poorly defined hypoechoic solid mass slightly taller than it is wide. Other suspicious nodules are seen as irregularly shaped hypoechoic masses with distal shadowing (Figure 8.45 [A]) or rounded, hypoechoic solid masses with microlobulated borders (Figure 8.46 [A]).

Correlating Ultrasonography and Mammography Findings

When an abnormality is detected on screening mammography, ultrasonography may subsequently

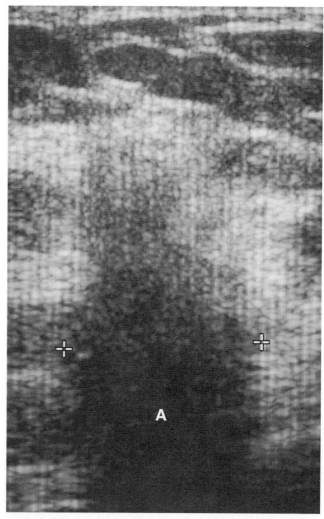

FIGURE 8.45

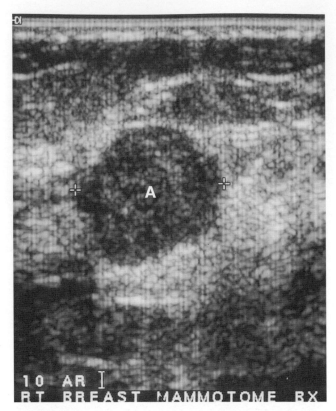

FIGURE 8.46

be performed. In these instances, the findings of the two examinations must be correlated to determine if the lesion detected on the mammogram corresponds to the sonographic findings. The correlation is necessary because multiple abnormalities may be present on both studies. Additionally mammography may detect abnormalities that were not seen during ultrasonography and vice versa.

The first determination is whether the mammographic and sonographic findings are located in the same portion of the breast. This correlation is usually straightforward. On occasion, however, it can be difficult, given that the breast is positioned differently for mammography and breast ultrasonography. If a question arises as to whether an abnormality seen on the two studies is the same, either mammographic or sonographic guidance can be used to place a radiopaque marker on the skin overlying the abnormality. The complementary study can then be performed to discover whether the abnormality seen and localized using the first modality corresponds in position to that seen using the second modality.

Lesion size must also be compared between the two modalities. On mammography, some magnifi-

cation of a lesion may occur as the distance of the lesion from the film screen detector increases. Some degree of consistency in the size of the abnormality as seen on the mammogram and the sonogram is required to ensure that the same lesion is being imaged.

Finally, the lesion characteristics seen on the two studies are compared. If mammography images a spiculated, irregular mass, ultrasonography should not image a cyst or a probably benign solid nodule. The expected finding of the sonogram would be an indeterminate or suspicious nodule.

MAGNETIC RESONANCE IMAGING OF THE BREAST
Evan Morton, MD

Magnetic resonance imaging (MRI) of the breast is an evolving modality that, as time passes, is most certain to play an increased role in the evaluation and management of breast pathology. Current limitations on the widespread use of MRI for breast pathology include issues of cost and availability; a lack of consensus on indications, imaging protocols, and interpretation of findings; and limited availability of devices that can be used in the MR suite for procedures to further evaluate abnormalities seen only on MRI examinations.

Current common uses of breast MRI are evaluating intracapsular and extracapsular rupture of breast implants and searching for a primary breast neoplasm in patients with metastatic disease to the axillary lymph nodes when mammography and ultrasonography have been negative. Some authors recommend the routine use of preoperative breast MRI for patients with DCIS or invasive malignancies. The MRI examination can evaluate the possibility that the disease is more extensive than can be appreciated mammographically and can search for mammographically occult multicentric or multifocal disease.

Breast MRI is currently performed using high field strength MRI units (1.0–1.5 T) with a dedicated breast coil. The patient is placed prone on the MR table with the breast in the dedicated coil. The patient is then placed into the bore of the MR magnet. When breast implant integrity is being evaluated, intravenous contrast is not used. When breast neoplasm is being evaluated, intravenous gadolinium is necessary.

Differentiating Benign and Malignant Lesions

No MRI protocol has been uniformly accepted for evaluating breast masses. Moreover, the various manufacturers have proprietary pulse sequences that may be common only to the scanners built by those manufacturers. However, most examiners feel that some form of T2 weighted image (such as a fast spin echo T2 weighted image) and a series consisting of one pre-gadolinium and multiple post-gadolinium enhanced rapidly acquired dynamic images (such as fast multiplanar spoil gradient images) should be used.

Unfortunately, no consensus has been reached on criteria for evaluating the significance of abnormalities seen on breast MRI images (that is, differentiating benign and malignant lesions). While the possibility of differences in the enhancement of breast parenchyma over the course of a woman's menstrual cycle are recognized, it is generally accepted that enhanced focal lesions represent pathology. However, the literature is divided concerning the findings that represent significant enhancement indicative of an abnormality requiring further investigation. Some authorities believe that lesion morphology is crucial; others believe that enhancement kinetics (that is, how the lesion enhances over time) are critical.

Examiners who feel that lesion morphology is paramount have emphasized the importance of ductal (linear) enhancement as suspicious for DCIS (Figure 8.47). However, the reported sensitivity of MRI in detecting DCIS has ranged from 40% to 100%.

In contrast, MRI detection of invasive carcinoma has been reported to approach 100%. The typical enhancement pattern of an invasive cancer is that of an enhancing, spiculated mass (Figure 8.48). Lesions with smooth or lobulated borders and internal septa that do not enhance, and masses with no enhancement have been reported to represent benign lesions.

The two most commonly encountered being benign lesions are cysts and fibroadenomas. Cysts that appear as round-to-ovoid smooth-bordered masses of high signal intensity on T2 weighted images and are of low signal intensity on T1 weighted images prior to intravenous gadolinium and do not enhance (Figure 8.49). Fibroadenomas can be seen as round-to-ovoid smooth-bordered masses, that enhance ho-

mogeneously and may have non-enhancing septation (Figure 8.50).

Examiners who believe that enhancement kinetics allow benign lesions to be distinguished from malignant ones have stressed the importance of time-versus-enhancement curves. In their scheme, lesions that enhance rapidly and "wash out" (demonstrate decreased enhancement soon after peak enhancement) over the course of a few minutes are felt to be highly suspicious. Lesions that enhance and fail to demonstrate a washout of contrast are felt to be benign.

Figure 8.47
A post-gadolinium fast multiplanar spoiled gradient recalled echo image (FMSPG) image demonstrates the ductal pattern of enhancement seen in ductal carcinoma in situ (DCIS).

Figure 8.48
Pre-dynamic (A) and post-dynamic (B) FMSPG images show invasive ductal carcinoma. In (A), the lesion is hypointense to the surrounding hyperintense fat and isointense to the fibroglandular tissue. In (B), the signal from fat is suppressed, and the lesion is seen as a spiculated area of enhancement (arrows).

Figure 8.49
Cysts are seen as areas of high signal intensity on T2 weighted images (A). On post-gadolinium enhanced T1 weighted FMSPG images (B), they are of low signal intensity and do not enhance.

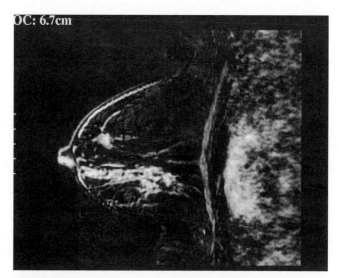

FIGURE 8.47

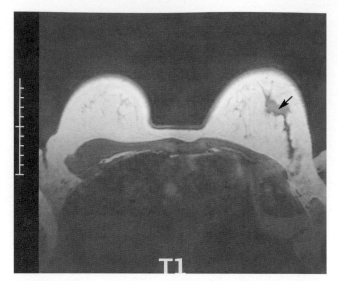

FIGURE 8.48A

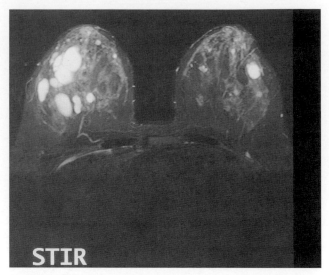

FIGURE 8.49A

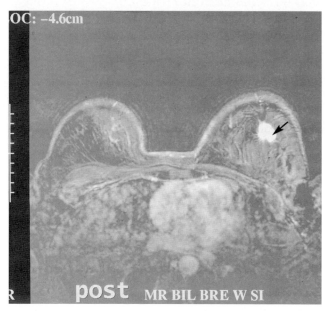

FIGURE 8.48B

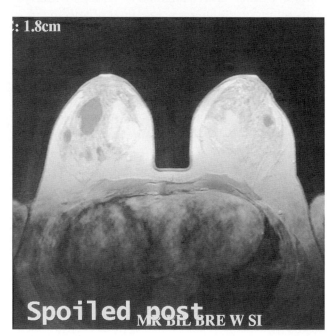

FIGURE 8.49B

Figure 8.50

A small fibroadenoma is imaged as a well-defined smooth-bordered area of enhancement on this post-gadolinium enhanced FMSPG image.

IMAGING OF BREAST IMPLANTS

Evaluation of breast implants for possible rupture is a well-established indication for breast MRI. The criteria for interpreting findings are also well established. An MRI of breast implants can determine not only if the implant is ruptured, but also the composition of the implant (silicone or saline), the structure of the implant (single-lumen or double-lumen), and the position of the implant (subglandular or subpectoral).

In evaluating for implant rupture, the examiner must first assess the integrity of the implant envelope. When the envelope is ruptured, it can be seen as a curvilinear line coursing through the fluid of the implant – a finding that has been called the "linguini sign" (Figure 8.51).

If implant envelope rupture has been established, then the type of rupture must be evaluated. That is to say, the examination must establish whether the rupture is intracapsular (the silicone or saline of the implant is contained by the fibrous capsule created by the body over time in response to the foreign substance, Figure 8.51) or extracapsular (the

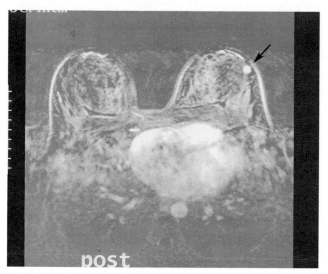

FIGURE 8.50

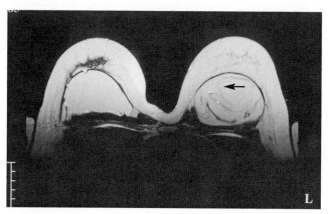

FIGURE 8.51

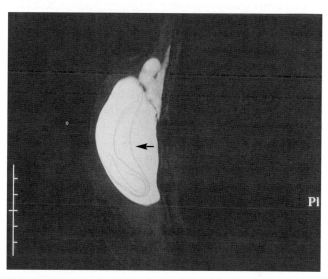

FIGURE 8.52

silicone or saline of the implant is outside the fibrous capsule surrounding the implant, Figure 8.52).

Figure 8.51
This MR image shows the "linguini sign" (arrow) in an intracapsular implant rupture of the left breast.

Figure 8.52
This MR image shows extracapsular implant rupture. Note "linguini" sign (arrow) and the presence of implant fluid (saline in this case) beyond the capsule (A).

INTERVENTION
EVAN MORTON, MD

NEEDLE LOCALIZATIONS

Before starting an open surgical biopsy for a nonpalpable breast lesion, a surgeon needs guidance to locate the mammographic or sonographic abnormality within the breast. Guidance ensures removal of the lesion while minimizing removal of surrounding normal tissue at surgery.

Various localization devices exist for the purpose of assisting the surgeon. In general, they work as described here. First, a hollow needle is placed into or directly adjacent to the lesion. Needle placement occurs under local anesthesia using mammo-

graphic, sonographic, or stereotactic guidance. Next, a wire that has a hook at its tip is inserted through the lumen of the needle. With some devices, the needle is then removed, and the wire, whose distal tip is anchored at the lesion, stays within the breast. The proximal end of the wire exits the skin. The surgical biopsy then proceeds, and the wire, with a variable amount of surrounding breast tissue, is removed (see chapter 10, "Role of the Surgeon – Biopsies").

To ensure adequate sampling of the lesion, an X-ray image of the removed tissue is taken. That image is called the specimen radiograph. If desired, speci-

mens that were localized preoperatively with ultrasound guidance can be examined sonographically after removal.

Mammography-Guided Needle Localization

To localize an abnormality using mammography guidance, the abnormality must be visualized in two orthogonal planes. Typically, the mediolateral oblique (MLO) or mediolateral (ML) projection and the cranial–caudal (CC) projection are used. The two planes provide the necessary information concerning depth of the lesion within the breast. An abnormality that is seen on only one mammographic view cannot be localized with mammography guidance. However, if the abnormality can be reproduced on a stereotactic device, the abnormality can be localized using that modality.

To localize an abnormality using mammography guidance, the breast is first placed in compression using a plate with a rectangular cutout at its center to accommodate the procedure. The sides of the cutout have radiopaque numbers along one side and radiopaque letters along the other. The cutout is arranged so that the lesion is within its confines, and the patient is usually positioned so that the needle will traverse the least amount of breast tissue in reaching the lesion during the localization.

A mammogram is then taken. The alphanumeric coordinates of the abnormality are noted on the mammogram, and the corresponding coordinates are marked on the patient's skin overlying the lesion.

Using sterile technique and local anesthesia, the localization needle is then placed into the breast while a light source simulates the path of the X-ray beam. To ensure that the tip of the needle is in the same plane as the lesion, the needle is placed so that it does not cast a shadow on the skin when the light source is on. Only the hub of the needle is visible as a shadow.

Mammograms are then taken in both planes with the needle in place. If the needle placement is satisfactory on those mammograms, the wire is then placed through the lumen of the needle. The needle is either withdrawn or left in place, depending on the type of localization device being used. If an adjustment to the needle position is necessary, that adjustment can be performed before the wire is deployed. (Some devices use a retractable wire, and adjustments can be made even after wire placement.)

Figure 8.53
Mammography-guided needle localization requires imaging two orthogonal planes. The lesion to

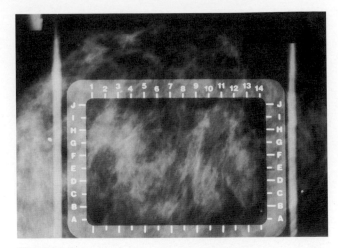

FIGURE 8.53A

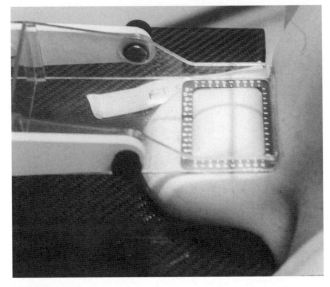

FIGURE 8.53B

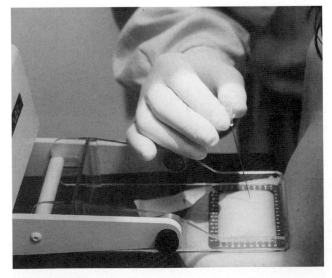

FIGURE 8.53C

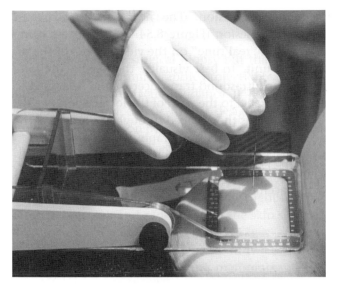

FIGURE 8.53D

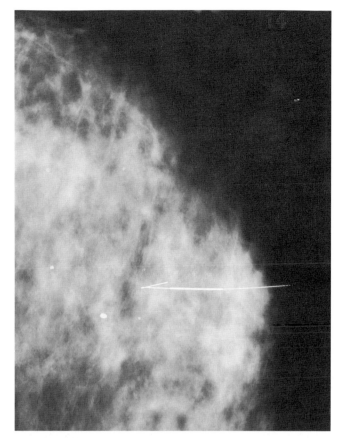

FIGURE 8.53F

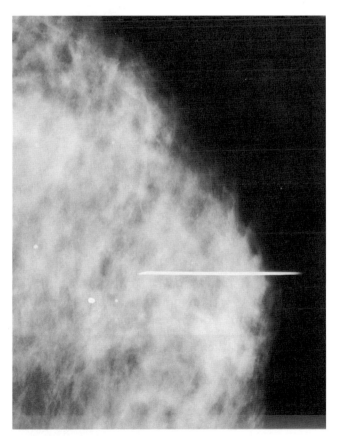

FIGURE 8.53E

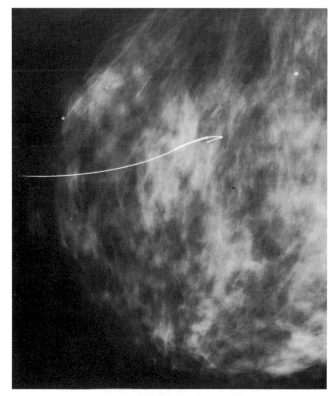

FIGURE 8.53G

be localized is placed within the confines of an alphanumeric grid (A). Crosshairs are aligned to overlie the abnormality (B). When needle placement is incorrect, the shadow of the needle projects onto the breast (C). When needle placement is correct, only the needle hub casts a shadow (D). The view orthogonal to that of the initial needle placement shows

9

Role of the Pathologist

SUSAN JORMARK, MD

The present chapter provides a basic pictorial introduction to breast pathology for the surgeon. It aims to assist him or her in understanding and visualizing the breast lesions discussed elsewhere in this book. Only the lesions most commonly encountered by a general pathologist are covered. For an in-depth discussion of breast pathology, including discussions of the more unusual breast diseases, readers are encouraged to consult textbooks on breast pathology (see Suggested Readings section).

OVERVIEW OF THE PATHOLOGIST'S ROLE

After physical examination reveals the presence of suspicious palpable lesions, or after mammography or other imaging studies reveal the presence of occult non-palpable abnormalities, a definitive diagnosis of cancer or benign breast disease rests with a histologic examination of the tissue. In addition to confirming the presence or absence of malignancy, the pathologist looks for morphologic features that help to predict the aggressiveness of a particular tumor, describes the extent and spread of disease, and indicates the adequacy of the surgical excision.

Pathologic features help to guide the surgeon, oncologist, and radiation therapist in planning therapy and in predicting prognosis. Morphology remains the most important pathologic feature in prognosis, but it is supplemented by important biologic, molecular, and genetic parameters that predict the behavior of a tumor and its response to various therapies. Examination of tissue may reveal lesions that, although still benign, increase the patient's risk of developing a malignancy. Various lesions confer various degrees of risk. Patients need to be followed carefully and may undergo various forms of prophylactic therapy.

The pathologist may receive for examination a specimen as small as a few cells aspirated with a fine needle or as large as a complete mastectomy with axillary lymph nodes (although the latter is much less common today). The most common pathology specimens are fine-needle aspirates, core biopsies, and lumpectomies (excision of the lesion with a margin of surrounding normal tissue). These specimens may serve both diagnostic and therapeutic functions, depending on the pathologic findings.

Tissue may be received during the course of surgery and quickly frozen by the pathologist for an immediate intraoperative diagnosis. That technique is most often used to establish adequacy of the excision, to determine the need for a complete dissection of axillary lymph nodes (by examination of the sentinel node), or simply to provide a rapid initial impression. Frozen-section diagnosis preceding mastectomy (in years past a common procedure) is now rarely performed.

INTERACTION OF THE SURGEON AND THE PATHOLOGIST

The manner in which the surgeon handles a specimen has an important bearing on the ability of the pathologist to make a complete and accurate diagnosis.

Labeling

Accurate labeling with complete relevant clinical history would seem too obvious to mention. However, the pathologist is, in fact, too often given insufficient information – or even worse, misinformation.

The patient's name and age and the specimen's side of origin (left or right) should be supplemented with information about prior studies (biopsies, fine-needle aspirations, previous excisions), prior treat-

ments (radiotherapy, chemotherapy), and relevant past and present medical history and medications. The fact that a mastectomy is being performed for prophylaxis should be indicated. If an excision is performed for microcalcifications, the specimen radiograph should be sent with the specimen.

One of the purposes of pathologic examination is to determine if a lesion has been entirely removed: that is, assessment of the excision margins. The edge of the tissue as seen on a glass slide is not necessarily the true site of excision. Ink placed on the outside surface of the gross specimen identifies the true margin (see chapter 12, "Surgical Treatment of Malignant Breast Lesions," Figure 12.25). The ink, visualized on the glass slide, indicates the true margin. If a specimen is incised before its arrival in pathology (by a curious surgeon who wants to see the lesion he has just removed), ink will seep into the cuts and crevices and will hinder accurate interpretation. Specimens must be sent to the laboratory whole and uncut.

If the surgeon feels it important to know not just whether a portion of tumor was left behind, but also where (medially, posteriorly, etc.) tumor was left behind (for the purpose of targeted re-excision), then the specimen must be oriented for the pathologist. Labeling should indicate whether the specimen comes from the right or left breast and should mark at least two of the three possible dimensional planes. For example, acceptable labeling could be anterior and medial, or posterior and lateral, or superior and lateral. Unacceptable labeling would be anterior and posterior, or medial and lateral, or superior and inferior. (See chapter 12, "Surgical Treatment of Malignant Breast Lesions," Figure 12.24.) The more detailed the labeling the better. The presence of a small piece of overlying skin indicates the anterior surface. In that case, only one other plane need be labeled by the surgeon. Using sutures as labels is better than using clips, because clips often fall off.

Surgeons often send separate pieces of tissue as margins. The pathologist receives the excision specimen and up to six additional specimens labeled by site. The surgeon must indicate on the margin specimen where the true new margin lies. Otherwise, the finding of tumor on the edge of the specimen may lead to the false impression that tumor still remains behind.

Frozen Sections

In the past, frozen-section examination of a breast lesion was followed by immediate mastectomy if the frozen section diagnosis indicated malignancy. That approach is only rarely taken today. Most frozen sections performed during breast surgery are requested by the surgeon simply to give the patient a rapid diagnosis (particularly if the lesion is benign). Intraoperative examination of a breast lesion is also performed to determine adequacy of the excision. Sentinel lymph nodes are frozen to determine the need for immediate axillary dissection. Many breast pathologists discourage the freezing of sentinel lymph nodes because much tissue is lost during preparation. Instead, they encourage the use of touch preparations to determine the presence of a metastatic tumor.

Some specimens should not or cannot be frozen. If a specimen is so small that freezing it amounts to freezing the entire specimen, and no residual unfrozen tissue remains for permanent sections, then the entire lesion will suffer from freezing artifact, which hampers interpretation. Freezing is particularly hazardous for in situ proliferative lesions of the breast. Diagnosis of in situ carcinomas and of hyperplasias, typical and atypical, and differentiation of those lesions one from another require excellent histology. For these reasons, specimens of non-palpable lesions (for example, microcalcifications) must not be frozen. Lesions only a few millimeters in diameter should not be frozen. Fat does not freeze well, and so highly fatty breast lesions cannot be frozen. A margin of normal fatty breast tissue around a tumor similarly does not freeze well. Intraoperative assessment of margins of excision therefore depends on gross examination rather than microscopic examination.

THE NORMAL FEMALE BREAST

Figure 9.1
The normal female breast consists of mammary lobules and ducts (A) in a fibro-fatty stroma (B).

Figures 9.2 and 9.3
The mammary lobule (Figure 9.2) is the secretory unit of the breast. It is composed of multiple acini. Secretory products (milk) in the acini enter intralobular ducts, exit the lobule through the terminal duct (see chapter 2, "Malignant Tumors," Figure 2.13), entering interlobular ducts of increasing diameter (Figure 9.3), and finally exit the breast through the major lactiferous ducts of the nipple.

The number of lobules is similar in all women, but the amount of fat and fibrous tissue in the breast

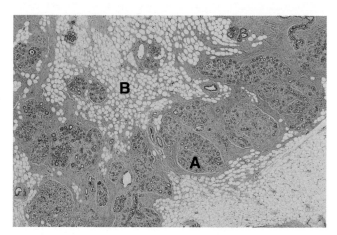

FIGURE 9.1

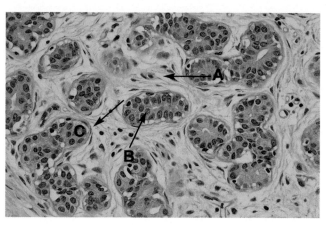

FIGURE 9.4

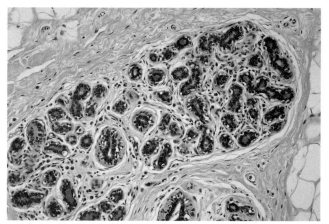

FIGURE 9.2

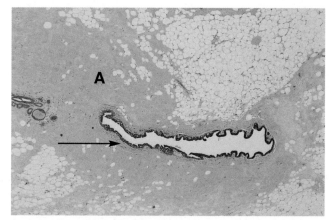

FIGURE 9.3

is highly variable. The male breast contains ducts, but rarely lobules.

Figure 9.4

The intralobular fibrous tissue is loose and may contain a sprinkling of inflammatory cells (Figure 9.4 [arrow A]). The interlobular fibrous tissue is more collagenous (see Figure 9.3[A]).

The lobular acinus is composed of an inner layer of cuboidal epithelial cells (arrow B) surrounded by an outer layer of myoepithelial cells, (arrow C) which is in turn surrounded by a basal lamina and basement membrane (seen with electron microscopy). The myoepithelial cells have contractile properties and help to expel the milk produced by the epithelial cells. (See chapter 2, "Malignant Tumors," Figure 2.14.)

Figure 9.5

The appearance of the lobule varies slightly during the various phases of the menstrual cycle. During pregnancy and lactation, under the influence of estrogens, progesterones, and prolactin, the epithelial cells enlarge and the cytoplasm becomes abundant, pale, and bubbly as milk production ensues.

Figures 9.6 and 9.7

The lobular acini become distended with secretory products, and the lobules and the breast as a

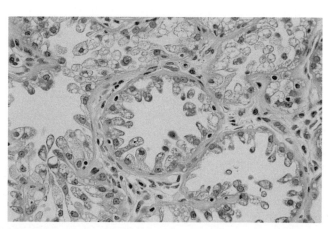

FIGURE 9.5

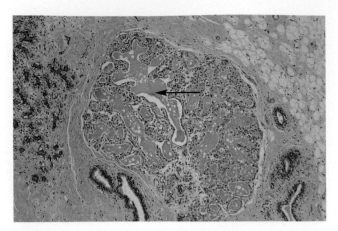

FIGURE 9.6

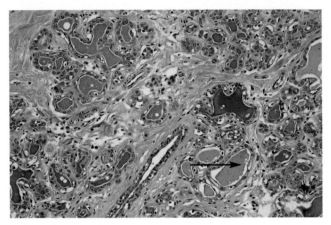

FIGURE 9.7

Fibrocystic change is characterized by several alterations in morphology that tend to occur together, each varying in extent, which may also occur in isolation. These alterations are collagenous fibrosis, cysts, apocrine metaplasia, adenosis,

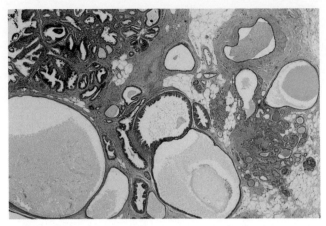

FIGURE 9.8

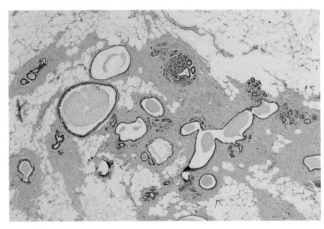

FIGURE 9.9

whole enlarge. In postmenopausal women the lobules atrophy.

COMMON BENIGN BREAST DISEASES

FIBROCYSTIC CHANGE

Fibrocystic change ("fibrocystic disease," "fibrocystic mastopathy") is the most common benign breast abnormality, being present to some extent in one third to one half of premenopausal women. The condition is believed to be a response to relative estrogen excess. It may be diffuse, patchy, or focal. It produces a well or poorly defined palpable lesion and is seen on mammography as an increase in density. Fibrocystic changes in the absence of proliferative features (discussed later in this chapter) or in the presence of only very mild ductal hyperplasia, does not in and of itself present a significant risk of future malignancy.

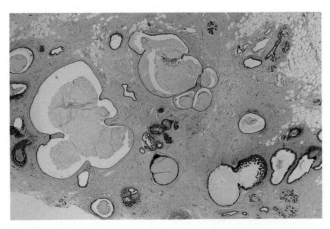

FIGURE 9.10

sclerosing adenosis, blunt duct adenosis, and mild ductal hyperplasia.

Figure 9.11

Collagenous fibrosis of the mammary stroma may be diffuse or patchy (imparting an overall dense firmness to the breast), or it may be focal or nodular (creating a discrete mass).

Figure 9.12

Cysts may be microscopic or large enough to create a palpable mass. Cysts are distended by a thin watery fluid and are lined by flattened ductal cells.

Figures 9.13 and 9.14

Apocrine metaplasia of the breast refers to replacement of the normal ductal epithelial cells by cells of the type seen in apocrine glands of the axillary skin (Figure 9.13). Apocrine cells have abundant pink granular cytoplasm and round nuclei, often with conspicuous nucleoli (Figure 9.14). Apocrine

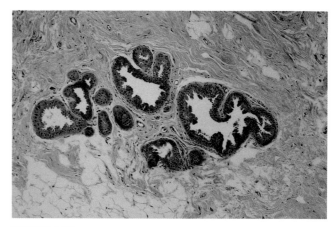

FIGURE 9.13

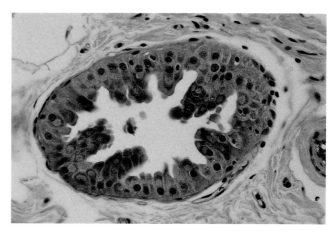

FIGURE 9.14

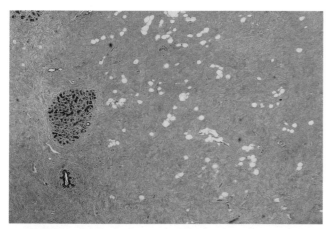

FIGURE 9.11

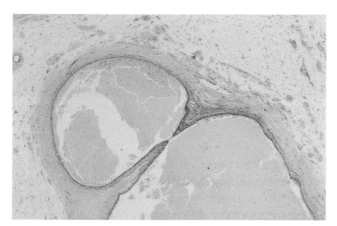

FIGURE 9.12

change is most often seen in benign ducts, with or without hyperplasia, but may be seen in lobules and may occur in malignancies.

Figures 9.15 and 9.16

In adenosis, the acini elongate and become tortuous so that the number of tubules appears increased on sectioning, and the lobule appears considerably enlarged (Figure 9.15). Lobules greatly enlarged by adenosis may appear to coalesce (Figure 9.16). Adenosis may become prominent enough to form a palpable mass called an "adenosis tumor."

Figures 9.17 and 9.18

In adenosis, fibrous-tissue proliferation may compress the tubules, reducing them to fine slits or obliterating them. The condition is called sclerosing adenosis, and it is seen more commonly in a slightly older age group. In sclerosing adenosis, the inner epithelial cell lining may atrophy, leaving behind only the spindled myoepithelial cells.

brous stroma (Figure 9.25) or may be associated with other benign lesions. Calcifications are also commonly found within the walls of blood vessels.

FIBROADENOMA

Fibroadenoma is the most common benign tumor. It usually arises in premenopausal patients.

Figures 9.26, 9.27, and 9.28

Fibroadenomas are multilobulated, but very well circumscribed (Figures 9.26 and 9.27). They are often very loosely attached to the surrounding breast tissue, enabling them to be shelled out (Figure 9.28).

Figures 9.29, 9.30, and 9.31

Fibroadenomas have both an epithelial and a fibrous stromal component. The fibrous stroma may proliferate within lobules, stretching and compressing the lobular epithelium (Figure 9.29), or it may grow around the lobular epithelium (Figure 9.30). The epithelial component may be simple or hyperplastic, and components of fibrocystic changes may be pres-

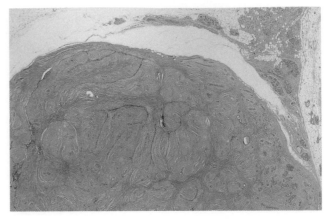

FIGURE 9.28

ent. In younger patients, the stroma is more cellular (Figure 9.31). Fibroadenomas with stromal hypercellularity need to be distinguished from phyllodes tumors.

Figures 9.32 and 9.33

Usually, fibroadenomas large enough to be palpated are removed. Small, clinically silent fibroade-

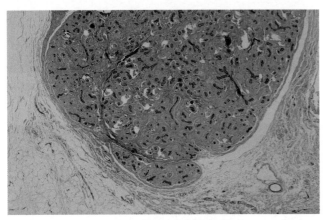

FIGURE 9.26

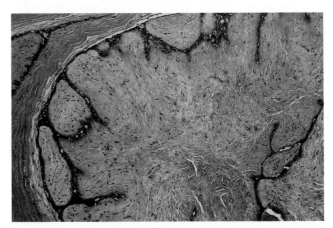

FIGURE 9.29

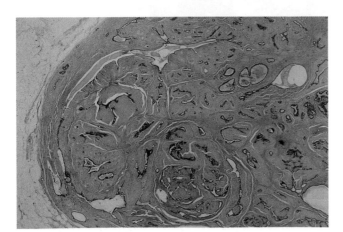

FIGURE 9.27

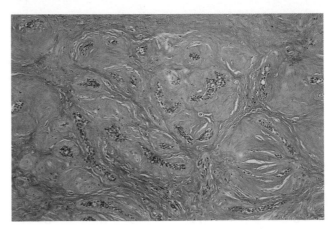

FIGURE 9.30

nomas that remain within the patient undergo hyalinization of the stroma as the patient ages (Figure 9.32). These fibroadenomas may be discovered incidentally in older women in tissue removed for other reasons, or they may come to medical attention because of the large, coarse calcifications that frequently form within them (Figure 9.33; also see chapter 1, "Benign Tumors," Figures 1.15 and 1.16). Complete removal of lesions that appear on core biopsy to be fibroadenomas is desirable, because phyllodes tumors may have components histologically identical to benign fibroadenomas.

PAPILLOMA

Papillomas are branching proliferations that grow within ducts. They may be solitary or multiple.

Figure 9.34

Solitary papillomas are more common. They usually grow within large, more centrally located ducts (often in major lactiferous ducts of the nipple), causing nipple discharge that may be bloody. (See chapter 4, "Symptoms of the Nipple-Aerola Complex," Figure 4.30.) Involved ducts frequently become cystically distended (intracystic papilloma).

Figures 9.35 and 9.36

Papillomas are characterized by branching fronds with fibrovascular cores (Figure 9.35). The fronds are covered by a dual layer of ductal epithelial cells (arrow A) and underlying myoepithelial cells (arrow B), as are normal ducts (Figure 9.36). The presence of myoepithelial cells distinguishes papillomas from papillary carcinomas, which lack that layer.

Figure 9.37

Papillomas may be quite complex. They may undergo sclerosis. Proliferative changes of the ductal epithelium, from hyperplasias to in situ carcinomas, may be superimposed.

Figure 9.38

Multiple papillomas (papillomatosis) tend to be smaller and more peripherally located. They are seen in the setting of fibrocystic change (Figure

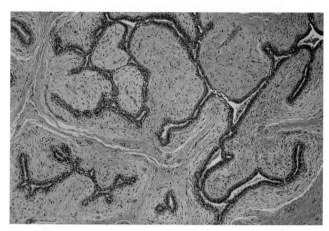

FIGURE 9.31

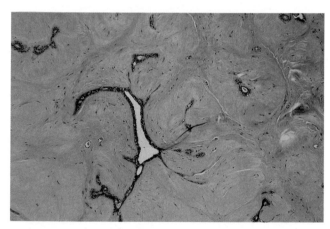

FIGURE 9.32

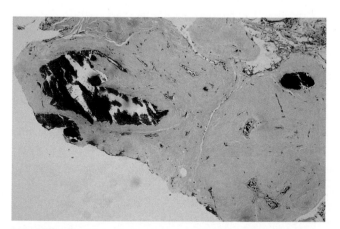

FIGURE 9.33

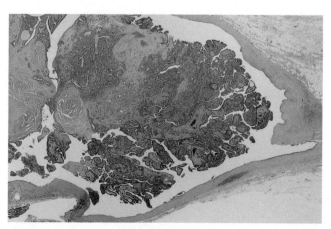

FIGURE 9.34

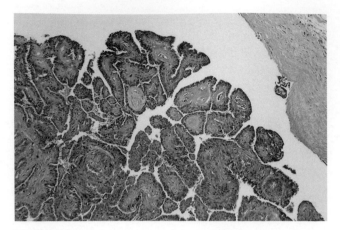

FIGURE 9.35

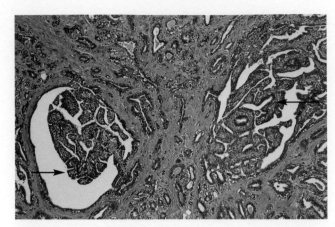

FIGURE 9.38

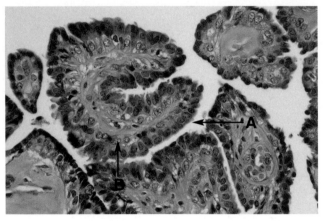

FIGURE 9.36

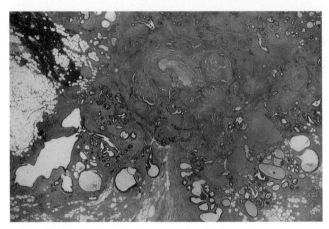

FIGURE 9.39

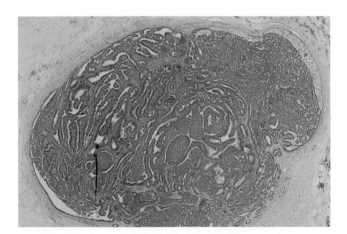

FIGURE 9.37

9.38). Papillomatosis is associated with a slightly higher risk of subsequent carcinoma than is solitary papilloma.

RADIAL SCAR

Radial scars occur when a focal fibroelastotic proliferation ("scar") pulls in and distorts the surround-

ing breast tissue, creating radiating tissue bands like the spokes of a wheel.

Figure 9.39

Radial scars may be solitary or multiple (Figure 9.39; also see chapter 8, "Role of the Radiologist," Figure 8.24). They are usually non-palpable and are detected by mammography. Their greatest significance lies in their radiologic appearance, which mimics that of an invasive carcinoma. Excision is required to differentiate them from tumor.

Figures 9.40 and 9.41

The central scar is composed of fibrous tissue and elastic tissue (Figure 9.40). The scar compresses epithelial structures, creating a pseudoinvasive appearance. The presence of myoepithelial cells around the ductules attests to their benign nature (Figure 9.41). The radiating bands, composed of distorted ducts and lobules, may show fibrocystic changes with or without proliferation of the ductal epithelium (for example, hyperplasia). The risk of

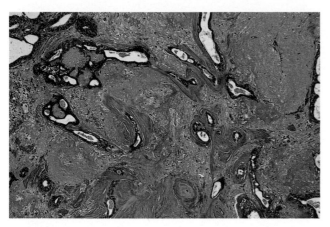

FIGURE 9.40

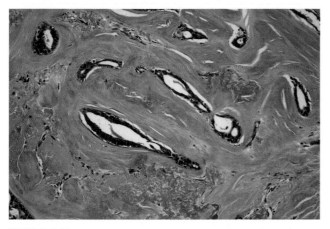

FIGURE 9.41

subsequent carcinoma in patients with radial scars depends on the presence and nature of the proliferative changes (just as in patients without radial scars). The presence of the "scar" in and of itself has no prognostic importance.

BREAST LESIONS CONFERRING SIGNIFICANT RISK OF SUBSEQUENT CARCINOMA

The breast lesions discussed in this subsection, although benign in themselves, are associated with a significantly greater risk to the patient of subsequent breast carcinoma than are the lesions discussed earlier in the chapter. These lesions – ordinary ductal hyperplasia, atypical ductal hyperplasia, atypical lobular hyperplasia, and lobular carcinoma in situ – do not, in and of themselves, necessarily become cancerous (that is, they are not pre-malignant). Instead, they indicate a tendency of the breast epithelium as a whole to undergo malignant change.

Risk may be expressed in various ways. One method is to describe relative risk – that is, the risk of developing cancer in members of a specific group, relative to the same risk in the general population. For example, a relative risk of 4× indicates a risk of developing cancer that is four times greater than the risk in the general population. The relative risk for a given lesion should not be taken out of context; it is influenced by the age of the patient, family history of breast carcinoma, and time interval after diagnosis.

The hyperplasias and lobular carcinoma in situ increase the risk of carcinoma globally: that is, in both breasts about equally. The lesions are microscopic, non-palpable, and generally not mammographically detectable. They are therefore discovered incidentally in breast tissue removed for other reasons.

ORDINARY DUCTAL HYPERPLASIA

Ductal hyperplasia of the ordinary type refers to an intraductal proliferation of the epithelial cells that line the duct, forming delicate cellular strands or tufts.

Ductal hyperplasia is frequently seen in the setting of fibrocystic changes. Ordinary ductal hyperplasia is associated with a relative risk of carcinoma of approximately 2×.

Figures 9.42 and 9.43
The strands of ductal hyperplasia may bridge the lumen to form a lacelike pattern or may fill the lumen to form solid or almost solid cellular growths, leaving behind only slit-like or irregularly shaped peripherally located spaces (Figure 9.42). The cells are typically slightly spindled. They vary somewhat in appearance and have overlapping nuclei, creating a haphazard, disheveled appearance (Figure 9.43).

Figure 9.44
Hyperplasias may be composed of apocrine cells.

ATYPICAL DUCTAL HYPERPLASIA

Atypical ductal hyperplasia is ductal hyperplasia with some, but not all, of the features of ductal carcinoma in situ. For low-grade ductal carcinoma in situ morphologic and quantitative criteria (size of duct or aggregate diameter of involved ducts) are both required for diagnosis. Quantitative criteria are not necessary for cytologically high-grade lesions. Atypical ductal hyperplasia falls short of the criteria for intraductal carcinoma either morphologically or quantitatively.

Atypical ductal hyperplasia confers a relative risk of carcinoma of approximately 4×–5×.

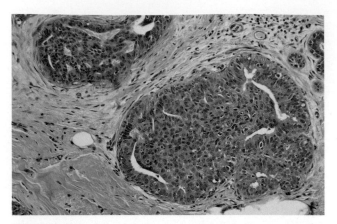

FIGURE 9.42

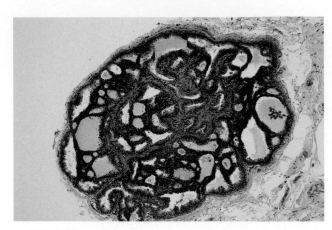

FIGURE 9.45

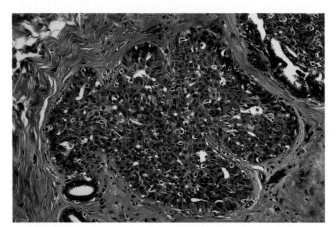

FIGURE 9.43

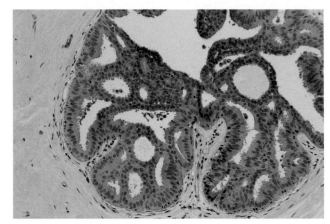

FIGURE 9.46

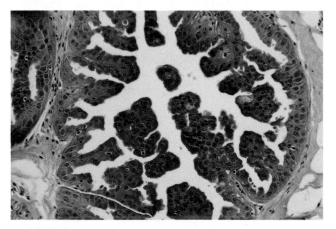

FIGURE 9.44

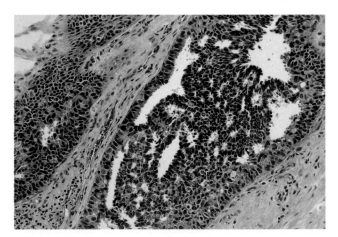

FIGURE 9.47

Figures 9.45, 9.46, 9.47, 9.48, and 9.49

The morphologic features of atypical ductal hyperplasia that mimic ductal carcinoma may be cytologic or architectural in nature. The atypical features include proliferations that form spaces that are round and centrally located (Figure 9.45), or that are composed of cells that are too uniform (Figure 9.46) or that have enlarged hyperchromatic nuclei with high nuclear/cytoplasmic ratios (Figure 9.47). Some atypical ductal hyperplasias are of the "flat" type, showing minimal intraluminal proliferation but significant cytologic

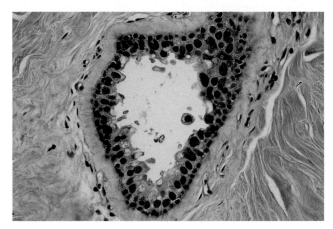

FIGURE 9.48

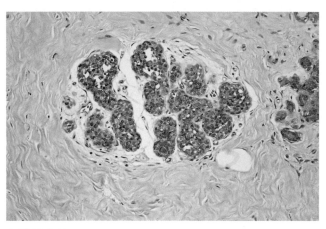

FIGURE 9.50

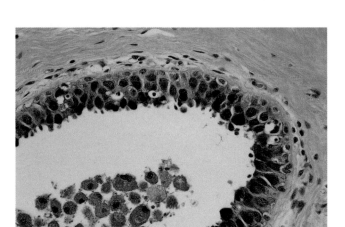

FIGURE 9.49

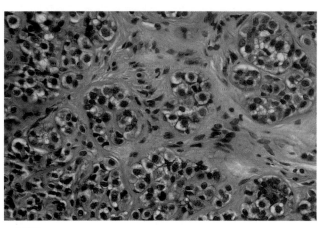

FIGURE 9.51

atypia (Figure 9.48). With sufficient cytologic atypia they may be considered to be "clinging" ductal carcinoma in situ (Figure 9.49), a lesion that is controversial.

ATYPICAL LOBULAR HYPERPLASIA

Atypical lobular hyperplasia refers to a proliferation of lobular-type cells within the acini of a lobule. It is part of the spectrum of lobular neoplasia, which encompasses atypical lobular hyperplasia and lobular carcinoma in situ. These two conditions differ primarily in the degree of proliferation.

Atypical lobular hyperplasia confers a relative risk of carcinoma of approximately 4×–5×.

Figures 9.50 and 9.51

In atypical lobular hyperplasia, the cellular proliferation is mild. The cells fill or partially fill the acini, but do not substantially distend most of them (Figure 9.50). The proliferating cells are small and have uniform, round nuclei (Figure 9.51).

LOBULAR CARCINOMA IN SITU

Lobular carcinoma in situ refers to a proliferation of lobular-type cells within acini (as in atypical lobular hyperplasia), but to a more significant degree.

Although the term "carcinoma" is used, this appellation is a misnomer, because the lesion is not considered a true malignancy or even pre-malignant. The lesion itself does not evolve into a carcinoma. Instead, it is a risk factor for the development of carcinoma.

Surgically removing all foci of lobular carcinoma in situ will not eliminate the risk. The condition confers a relative risk of approximately 9×–11×, and the increased risk applies to both breasts equally. Most carcinomas arising in the setting of lobular carcinoma in situ are of the ductal type. Approximately one third are of infiltrating lobular type.

Figures 9.52 and 9.53

In lobular carcinoma in situ most acini in a lobule are solidly filled and distended by proliferating

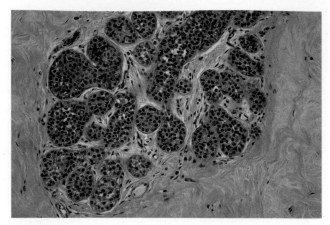

FIGURE 9.52

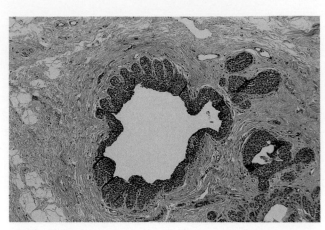

FIGURE 9.54

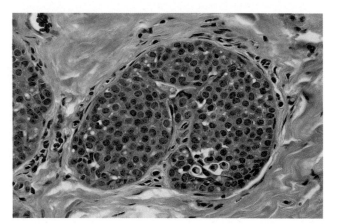

FIGURE 9.53

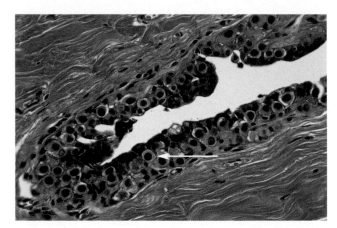

FIGURE 9.55

cells of lobular carcinoma in situ type (Figure 9.52). The cells are small, with uniform, round nuclei (Figure 9.53). Small spaces may be created between the cells owing to lack of cohesion.

Figures 9.54, 9.55, and 9.56

The cells of lobular carcinoma in situ may extend into ducts, creating a cloverleaf pattern around the duct (Figure 9.54). They spread in a so-called page-toid manner between the native epithelial cells that line the duct and the outer myoepithelial cells (Figure 9.55) (arrow). In some instances, the degree of proliferation is so great as to obliterate the normal underlying acinar architecture (Figure 9.56).

DUCTAL CARCINOMA IN SITU AND MICROINVASIVE CARCINOMA

Ductal carcinoma in situ (intraductal carcinoma) is a proliferation of fully malignant cells at a very

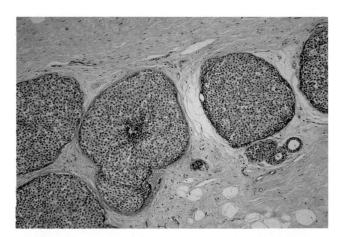

FIGURE 9.56

early stage, when the cells are still within the duct, before they have invaded the surrounding fibro-fatty stroma. They are still separated from the stroma by the basal lamina (visualized by electron microscopy). By light microscopy, the involved ducts are usually surrounded by a layer of myoepithelial cells. Because

the stroma has not yet been penetrated, the malignant cells do not yet have access to blood vessels and lymphatics. They thus cannot metastasize. As a result, complete surgical resection is curative.

In contrast to those proliferative lesions that indicate increased risk for developing carcinoma at sites other than the foci of proliferation, ductal carcinoma in situ, in and of itself, may evolve into invasive carcinoma if not eliminated. Ductal carcinoma in situ may (but most often does not) form a palpable mass. Hence, it may go undetected until invasion occurs.

Important to the diagnosis of ductal carcinoma in situ in its curative stage is the mammographic detection of microcalcifications. Microcalcifications occur in a significant proportion of intraductal carcinomas, approximately 75%–95% (see chapter 8, "Role of the Radiologist," Figures 8.14 through 8.20).

Grade and Pattern

Ductal carcinoma in situ is categorized according to grade (low, intermediate, high) and pattern (cribriform, solid, comedo, micropapillary, papillary). Grade is more significant than pattern.

While no universally accepted grading system exists, most breast pathologists grade according to nuclear features. They may or may not consider the presence or absence of central necrosis.

Figure 9.57
Low-grade (grade 1) lesions of ductal carcinoma in situ have cell nuclei that are small, round, and uniform.

Figure 9.58
Grade 2 lesions of ductal carcinoma in situ have nuclei that are larger and more variable in size and shape.

Figure 9.59
Grade 3 lesions of ductal carcinoma in situ have nuclei that are large, irregular, more pleomorphic (variable in appearance), and often hyperchromatic.

Figures 9.60 and 9.61
The cribriform pattern of ductal carcinoma in situ is characterized by intraluminal formation of round, centrally located, gland-like spaces and bridging arches.

Figure 9.62
The solid pattern of ductal carcinoma in situ refers to the solid filling of ducts by the cells.

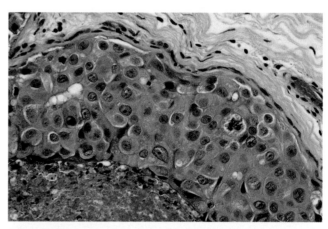

FIGURE 9.58

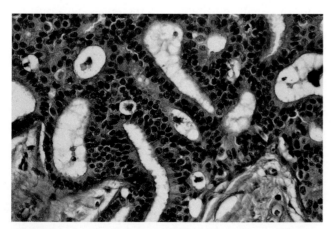

FIGURE 9.57

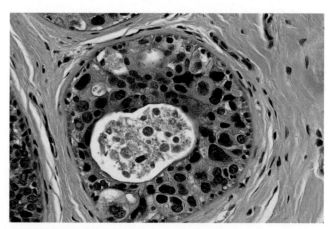

FIGURE 9.59

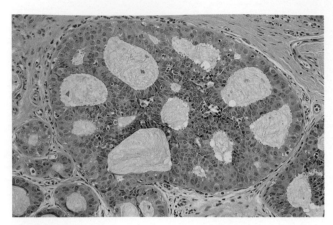

FIGURE 9.60

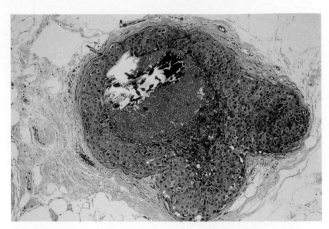

FIGURE 9.63

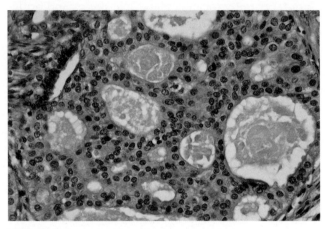

FIGURE 9.61

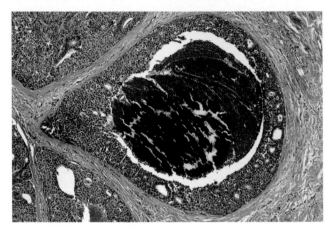

FIGURE 9.64

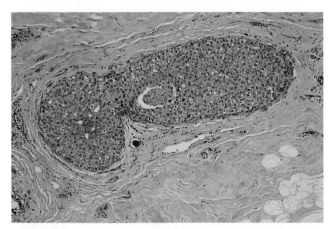

FIGURE 9.62

Figures 9.63 and 9.64

The comedo pattern of ductal carcinoma in situ refers to a combination of high nuclear grade and central necrosis. The necrosis may be so extensive that, grossly, the necrotic material may be expressed from the lumen as in a comedone (see chapter 2, "Malignant Tumors," Figure 2.15). Central necrosis

may also be seen in lower grade intraductal carcinoma. Calcification occurs in the central necrotic area and can be seen mammographically.

Figures 9.65, 9.66, and 9.67

The micropapillary pattern refers to the formation of small epithelial excrescences without fibrovascular cores. These project into the duct lumen (Figures 9.65 and 9.66). The micropapillary fronds may fuse creating an appearance overlapping with that of the cribriform pattern (Figure 9.67).

Figures 9.68, 9.69, and 9.70

The papillary pattern demonstrates branching fronds with fibrovascular cores. The involved duct may become cystically dilated, creating an intracystic papillary carcinoma (Figure 9.69). Papillary carcinoma greatly resembles the benign papilloma; however, the fronds in the papilloma are covered by a dual layer of epithelial cells and myoepithelial cells (Figure 9.36). In papillary carcinoma, the fronds are

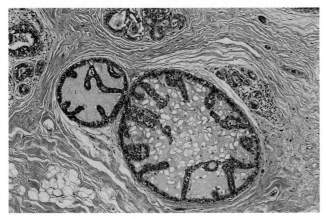

FIGURE 9.65

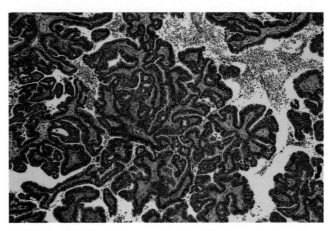

FIGURE 9.68

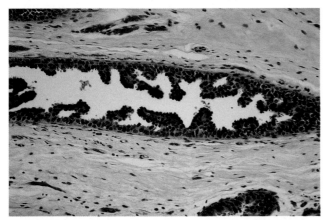

FIGURE 9.66

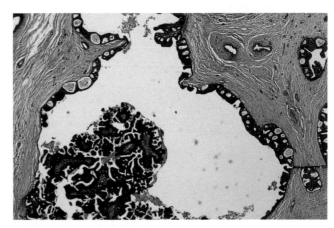

FIGURE 9.69

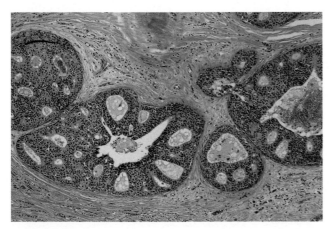

FIGURE 9.67

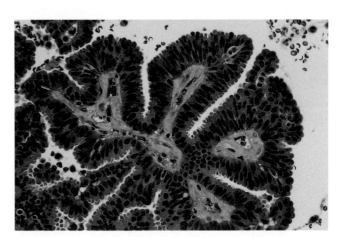

FIGURE 9.70

covered by epithelial cells without a myoepithelial cell layer (Figure 9.70).

Figures 9.71 and 9.72

Just as the lobular cells of lobular carcinoma in situ spread into the duct, so may the ductal cells of ductal carcinoma in situ spread into lobules, re-placing the normal cell population. This process is known as retrograde cancerization of the lobules. The cells are still limited to the epithelium. They are bounded by myoepithelial cells and basal lamina and basement membrane, and are therefore still in situ.

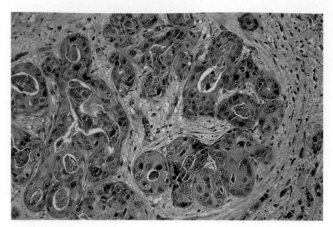

FIGURE 9.71

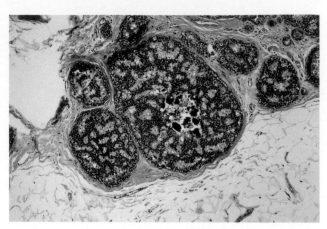

FIGURE 9.73

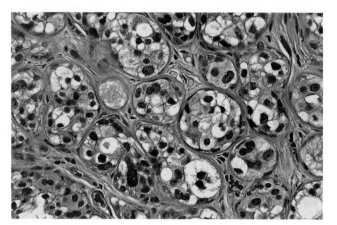

FIGURE 9.72

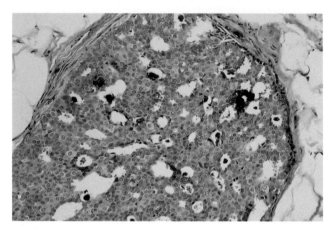

FIGURE 9.74

Figures 9.73, 9.74, and 9.75

As previously mentioned, ductal carcinoma in situ frequently has associated microcalcifications. The calcifications are largest and most frequent in comedo necrosis (see Figures 9.63 and 9.64), but they may be seen in any pattern of intraductal carcinoma with or without necrois (Figures 9.73, 9.74, and 9.75). The discovery of small or in situ carcinomas by detection of their associated microcalcifications is one of the most important benefits of mammography.

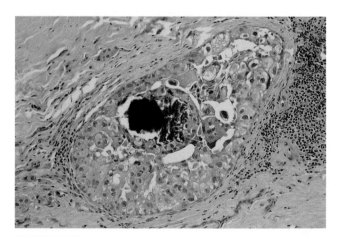

FIGURE 9.75

Microinvasive Carcinoma

Microinvasive ductal carcinoma is the very earliest stage of stromal invasion. "Micro" refers to foci of invasion no larger than 1 mm in size. Because malignant cells have penetrated the basal lamina and basement membrane and entered the stroma, they do in theory have the potential to reach blood vessels and lymphatics, and hence to metastasize. In practice, however, invasive carcinoma of this extremely small size has been found to behave like carcinoma in situ. Several foci of invasion may be present in a patient; as long as each separate focus is no larger than 1 mm, the lesion is still considered to be microinvasive.

Figures 9.76, 9.77, and 9.78

Microinvasion may be seen as a small tongue of cells projecting into the surrounding stroma (Figure 9.76 [arrow]). It may consist of no more than a few malignant cells in a reactive desmoplastic stroma (Figures 9.77 [arrow] and 9.78). Microinvasive carci-

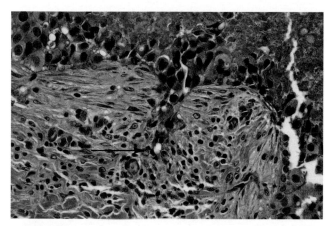

FIGURE 9.76

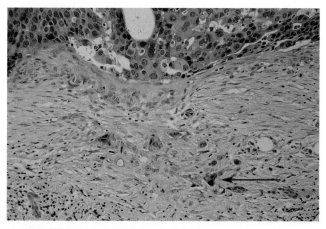

FIGURE 9.77

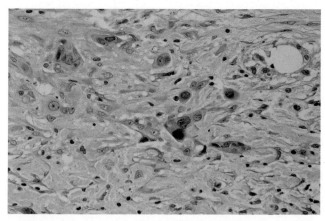

FIGURE 9.78

noma is associated more commonly with high-grade comedo intraductal carcinoma.

INVASIVE CARCINOMA AND OTHER MALIGNANT TUMORS

Only the most common forms of breast carcinoma and phyllodes tumor are covered here. Discussion of unusual carcinoma types, various sarcomas (other than phyllodes tumor), lymphomas, and metastases to the breast from other sites can be found in textbooks on breast pathology.

The two most common carcinoma types are infiltrating ductal and infiltrating lobular carcinoma. Variants of ductal carcinoma that are much less common but not extraordinarily rare are tubular carcinoma, colloid (mucinous) carcinoma, medullary carcinoma, papillary carcinoma, and cribriform carcinoma. Inflammatory carcinoma and Paget's disease are not specific tumor types but unusual presentations. (See chapter 2, "Malignant Tumors," Figures 2.17 through 2.31.)

Every carcinoma type may be graded. Some tumor types are essentially always low grade (for example, tubular carcinoma, colloid carcinoma), and some are always high grade (for example, medullary carcinoma). Other tumor types show variable grades. The most commonly accepted grading system is the modified Scarff–Bloom–Richardson system. It uses a point system based on architecture, nuclear features, and mitotic activity. Total points may range from 3 to 9, categorizing the carcinoma into grades 1, 2, or 3 (low, intermediate, or high).

Tumor type, tumor grade, tumor size, extent of local invasion, presence or absence of lymphatic or distant metastases, and biologic markers (estrogen and progesterone receptors, DNA ploidy, S-phase fraction, and HER-2/*neu*) are used to determine prognosis and treatment. (More detail is provided later in this chapter.)

On gross inspection, most carcinomas are firm, gritty, stellate nodules firmly attached to the surrounding breast tissue. Some carcinomas may, however, be unusually well circumscribed (for example, colloid carcinomas and medullary carcinomas). Conversely, some carcinomas may not form discrete nodules; they infiltrate the breast diffusely in a non-circumscribed fashion (for example, lobular carcinoma). Colloid carcinomas tend to be softer, mucoid, and glistening; medullary carcino-

mas are softer and fleshy; lobular carcinomas may mimic fat necrosis.

INFILTRATING DUCTAL CARCINOMA

Infiltrating ductal carcinoma is the most common type of invasive carcinoma, accounting for 50%–60% of breast carcinomas in women and 85% of breast carcinomas in men.

Figures 9.79 and 9.80
Infiltrating ductal carcinoma has irregular microscopic borders.

Figures 9.81, 9.82, and 9.83
Infiltrating ductal carcinoma is characterized by the formation of ductules or tubules with distinct lumens. The percentage of the tumor in which ductule formation is seen constitutes the degree of architectural differentiation (architectural grade). Tubule formation may be good (Figure 9.81), intermediate (Figure 9.82), or poor (Figure 9.83).

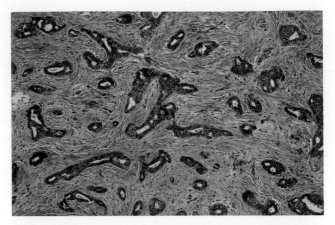

FIGURE 9.81

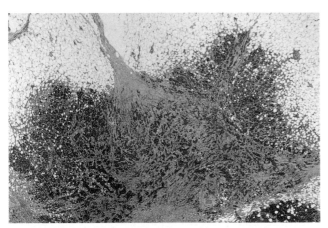

FIGURE 9.79

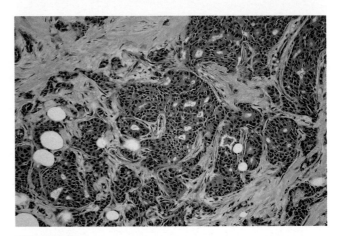

FIGURE 9.82

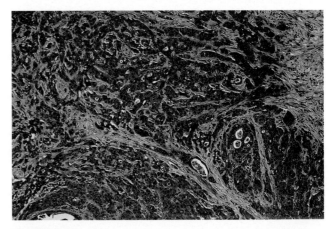

FIGURE 9.83

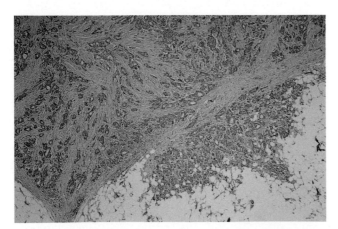

FIGURE 9.80

Figures 9.84, 9.85, and 9.86
Nuclei of infiltrating ductal carcinoma cells are graded in a way similar to that used to grade intraductal carcinoma: low grade (Figure 9.84), intermediate grade (Figure 9.85), or high grade (Figure 9.86).

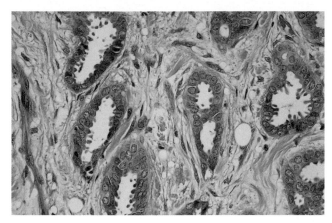

FIGURE 9.84

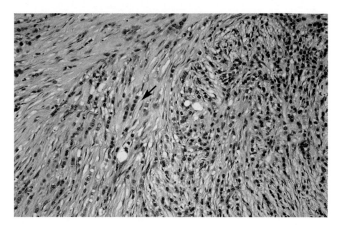

FIGURE 9.87

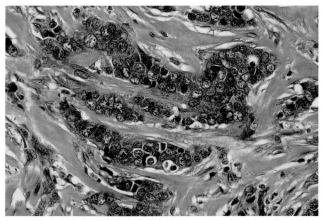

FIGURE 9.85

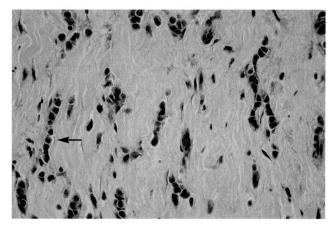

FIGURE 9.88

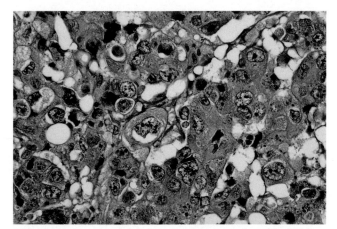

FIGURE 9.86

INFILTRATING LOBULAR CARCINOMA

Infiltrating lobular carcinoma has several variants (classic, solid, alveolar, tubulolobular, signet ring, histiocytoid, apocrine, pleomorphic, and mixed), but it does not form ductules. The overall long-term prognosis for classic infiltrating lobular

carcinoma is similar to that for infiltrating ductal carcinoma, but varies somewhat with grade and subtype.

Figures 9.87 and 9.88

The cells of infiltrating lobular carcinoma infiltrate most commonly in very delicate single files called Indian files (Figure 9.87 and 9.88, arrows), although other patterns may be seen.

Figures 9.89 and 9.90

The cells of infiltrating lobular carcinoma tend to have small and uniform nuclei and scant cytoplasm (Figure 9.89), but they may have larger, more pleomorphic nuclei (pleomorphic variant, Figure 9.90).

Figure 9.91

Although infiltrating lobular carcinomas may be as circumscribed as infiltrating ductal carcinomas, they frequently are not. Sometimes they create a diffuse, poorly defined region of induration involving a large portion of the breast. Often, a rela-

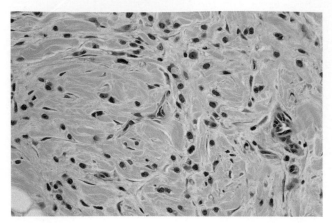

FIGURE 9.89

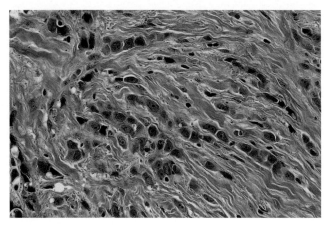

FIGURE 9.90

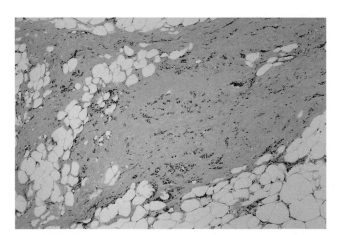

FIGURE 9.91

tively small number of tumor cells invade surrounding normal tissue insidiously (Figure 9.91), rendering accurate gross evaluation of tumor margins impossible.

TUBULAR CARCINOMA

Tubular carcinoma is a particularly well differentiated (low grade) variant of infiltrating ductal carcinoma.

Figures 9.92 and 9.93

The ductules of tubular carcinoma have wide-open lumens (Figure 9.92) and are lined with cells that are very low grade. The lining cells may have small cytoplasmic protrusions called apical snouts (Figure 9.93). The tumors tend to be small and may be multifocal. The rate of lymph node metastasis is lower with tubular carcinoma than with the ordinary ductal type. The overall prognosis is favorable.

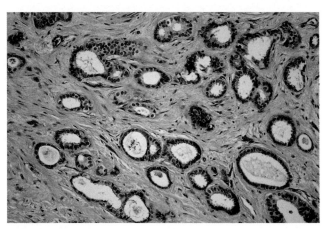

FIGURE 9.92

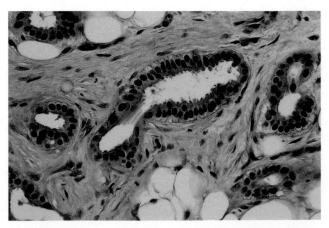

FIGURE 9.93

MUCINOUS CARCINOMA

Mucinous carcinoma is also known as colloid carcinoma.

Figures 9.94, 9.95, and 9.96

Mucinous carcinoma tumors are well circumscribed (Figure 9.94). They are characterized by abundant extracellular mucin (Figure 9.95 [arrow]),

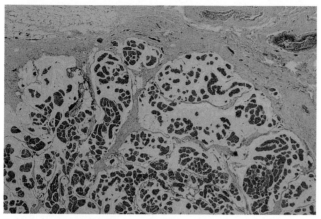

FIGURE 9.94

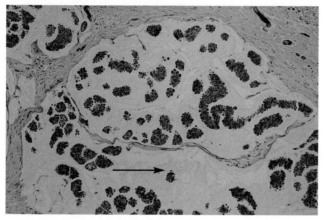

FIGURE 9.95

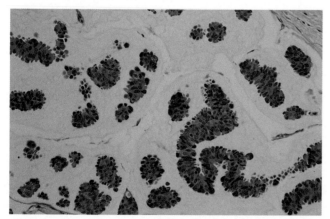

FIGURE 9.96

within which the tumor cells seem to float. The tumor cells are cytologically low grade (Figure 9.96). This tumor has a favorable prognosis.

MEDULLARY CARCINOMA

Medullary carcinoma has become considerably less common as the criteria for its diagnosis have become more stringent.

This tumor was previously thought to carry a favorable prognosis. Though some controversy exists, the tumor now appears to have a better prognosis than grade 3 (high-grade) ductal carcinomas, but no better prognosis than lower grade ductal carcinomas.

Figures 9.97 and 9.98

A medullary carcinoma tumor is well circumscribed (Figure 9.97) and contains an abundance of chronic inflammatory cells around the tumor periphery and between tumor cells (Figure 9.98). The tumor

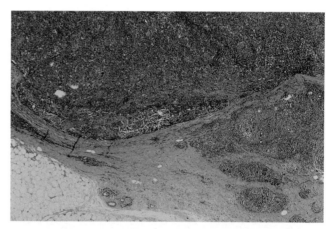

FIGURE 9.97

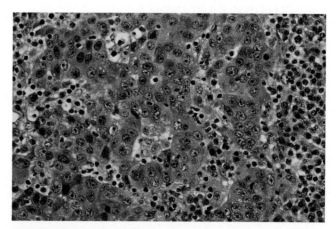

FIGURE 9.98

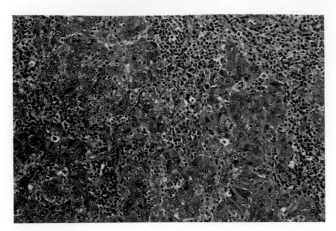

FIGURE 9.99

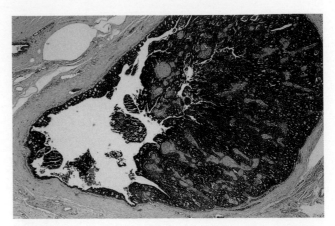

FIGURE 9.100

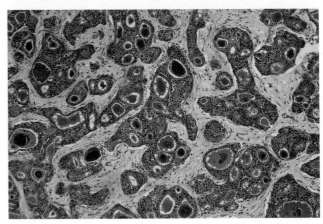

FIGURE 9.101

cells are large with large, vesicular nuclei and prominent nucleoli (Figure 9.98).

Figure 9.99
A medullary carcinoma does not form ductules, but instead is characterized by a syncytial sheet of cells.

PAPILLARY CARCINOMA

Figure 9.100
Most of the lesions called papillary carcinomas are actually still in situ or intracystic (Figure 9.100; also see Figures 9.68 through 9.70). When papillary carcinomas invade, they do so as ordinary ductal carcinomas. One exception is the rare micropapillary variant. Papillary carcinomas may have the florid branching frond pattern illustrated previously (see Figure 9.68), or they may have a more solid appearance owing to further proliferation of the epithelial cells or fibrous sclerosis.

CRIBRIFORM CARCINOMA

Figure 9.101
Cribriform carcinoma is characterized by infiltrating nests of tumor cells that form lumens similar to those seen in cribriform ductal carcinoma in situ (Figure 9.101). The tumor is low grade and has a good prognosis.

INFLAMMATORY CARCINOMA

Inflammatory carcinoma is not a particular tumor type, but a ductal carcinoma, usually high grade, accompanied by a reddened, inflammatory appearance of the overlying skin.

Inflammatory carcinoma requires particularly aggressive management. Patients are usually treated with chemotherapy before surgery.

Figures 9.102 and 9.103
In inflammatory carcinoma, histologic examination of the skin often, but not always, reveals tumor thrombi in the dermal lymphatics (Figure 9.102 and 9.103, arrows). The finding of dermal tumor thrombi alone, in the absence of a clinically inflamed appearance, is also considered to be inflammatory carcinoma. Thus, the diagnosis is made either clinically or through the pathologically.

PAGET'S DISEASE

Paget's disease of the nipple is also not a specific tumor type. The condition is a secondary spread of tumor cells into the epidermis of the nipple from an underlying carcinoma.

Paget's disease has no influence on prognosis in and of itself; prognosis depends on the nature and extent of the underlying tumor.

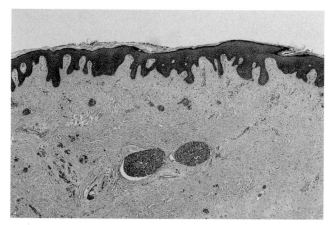

FIGURE 9.102

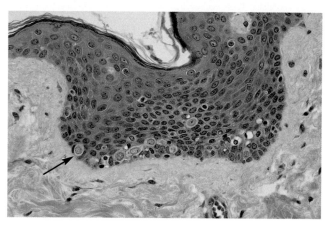

FIGURE 9.104

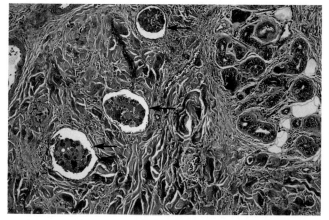

FIGURE 9.103

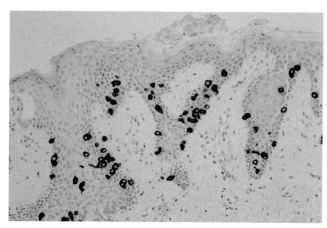

FIGURE 9.105

Figures 9.104 and 9.105

The major lactiferous ducts of the nipple are lined with the same double layer of inner ductal cells and outer myoepithelial cells as ducts elsewhere. As the ducts approach the surface, they become lined with squamous epithelium in continuity with the epidermis of the skin. Tumor cells of ductal carcinoma in situ within these ducts migrate up into the squamous lining and then into the overlying epidermis. The cells, usually lying at the base of the epidermis (Figure 9.104 [arrow]), are still in situ but may secondarily invade the underlying dermis. Special stains highlight the scattered tumor cells within the epidermis (Figure 9.105).

The underlying carcinoma in Paget's disease may be intraductal carcinoma only, but often is an invasive tumor. Paget's disease, clinically presenting as nipple changes, may be the first manifestation of a carcinoma (see chapter 2, "Malignant Tumors," Figures 2.17 through 2.21).

Metastasis and Recurrence

In addition to tumor type, size, and grade, the pathologist also examines resected breast tissue for evidence of invasion in the mammary blood vessels and lymphatic vessels, assesses completeness of the tumor resection, examines axillary lymph nodes for evidence of tumor metastases, and examines the surrounding breast tissue.

Figures 9.106 and 9.107

The presence of tumor thrombi within mammary lymphatics (Figure 9.106 and 9.107) correlates imperfectly with the presence of axillary lymph node metastases; however, when numerous mammary lymphatics are involved, the lymph nodes most often harbor tumor.

The presence of ductal carcinoma in situ in the surrounding breast tissue indicates a risk of tumor recurrence after limited resection.

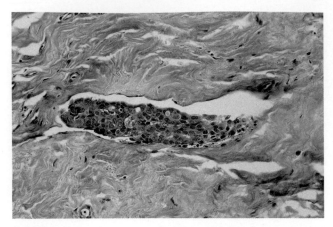

FIGURE 9.106

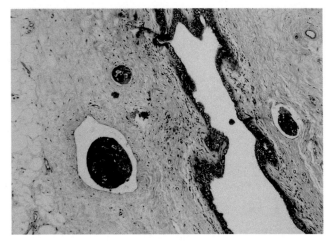

FIGURE 9.107

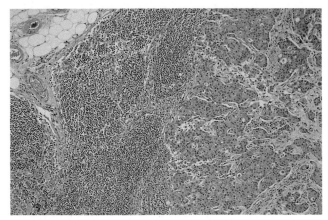

FIGURE 9.108

Figure 9.108

In the past, every breast resection for carcinoma was accompanied by removal of the corresponding axillary lymph nodes for both therapeutic and prognostic purposes. The pathologist would report the number of lymph nodes harboring tumor metastases (Figure 9.108). But axillary dissection is associated with significant morbidity. More recently, the surgeon initially removes only the lymph node that is the first to receive drainage from the breast (called the sentinel lymph node). If the sentinel node is negative for tumor, it is highly unlikely that the remaining nodes will be positive. Patients may therefore be spared a full axillary dissection.

Figure 9.109

Surgeons usually send the sentinel lymph node to the pathologist for immediate intraoperative examination, and the decision to remove the remaining lymph nodes is made at the time of first surgery. If the sentinel lymph node is initially negative for tumor, the pathologist will later search the node more fully for occult micrometastasis by examining deeper levels of the node and by using special staining techniques (staining for cytokeratin by immunohistochemistry) to detect metastases of one or a few cells [Figure 9.109 (arrow)].

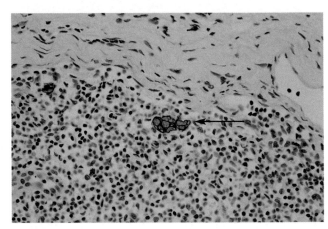

FIGURE 9.109

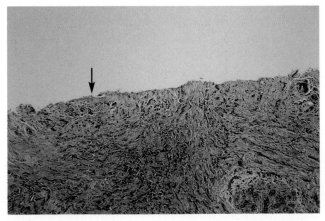

FIGURE 9.110

Figure 9.110

Because it is important that the surgeon remove the entire local tumor, the pathologist will examine the lines of resection (the margins) for presence of tumor. To identify the margins on the slide, the pathologist places ink on the exterior of the specimen. On a glass slide, the presence of tumor on the inked edge of the tissue (Figure 9.110) indicates the presence of tumor at the margin and hence incomplete resection of the tumor (arrow).

The pathologist may use varying colors of ink to color code the various margins (posterior, lateral, superior, etc.) if the surgeon situates the specimen for the pathologist, usually with the use of sutures.

Phyllodes Tumor

The only non-carcinomatous malignant neoplasm that will be discussed here is phyllodes tumor ("cystosarcoma phyllodes"). A phyllodes tumor is a fibroepithelial neoplasm similar to a fibroadenoma. In a phyllodes tumor, the stromal component undergoes a spectrum of malignant changes that range from low grade (benign phyllodes tumor) through intermediate grade to high grade (malignant phyllodes tumor). The epithelial component is benign.

The so-called benign phyllodes tumor does not usually metastasize, but if often recurs if incompletely resected. When it recurs, it may recur in a higher grade or as malignant phyllodes tumor. Malignant phyllodes tumor will metastasize in approximately one quarter of cases.

Figure 9.111

Phyllodes tumor is named for its leaf-like *(phyllodes)* appearance.

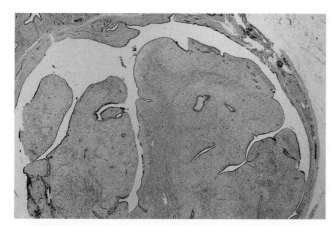

FIGURE 9.111

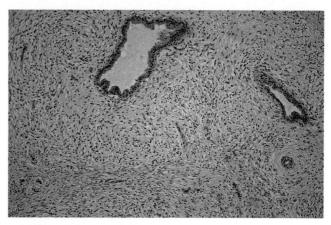

FIGURE 9.112

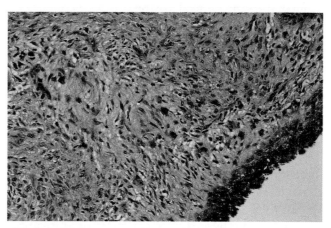

FIGURE 9.113

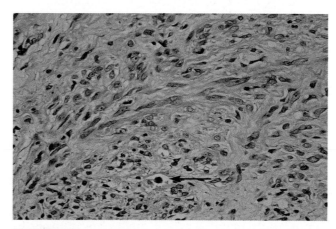

FIGURE 9.114

Figures 9.112, 9.113, and 9.114

Compared with a fibroadenoma, a phyllodes tumor contains more abundant stroma and exhibits greater cellularity (Figure 9.112), cytologic atypia (Figure 9.113), and mitotic activity (Figure 9.114 [arrow]).

Prognostic and Predictive Factors in Invasive Carcinoma

Prognostic factors pertain to the behavior of untreated carcinomas and hence to the overall survival of the patient. Predictive factors pertain to the response of tumors to specific treatments.

Some prognostic and predictive information is obtained by a standard assessment of morphology: tumor size, tumor type, tumor grade, lymph node metastases, and so on. Obtaining other prognostic and predictive information requires special techniques: hormone receptors, tumor proliferation rate, DNA ploidy, and oncogenes. Many potential factors are still under investigation and are not routinely evaluated in the clinical setting.

PROGNOSTIC FACTORS

The single best prognostic factor is the presence or absence of **metastases to axillary lymph nodes.** Survival is directly correlated with the number of nodes involved. The greater the number of lymph nodes harboring metastatic tumor, the poorer the patient's survival.

The size of the metastases also plays a role; metastases 2 mm or smaller are termed micrometastases. They have considerably less effect on survival than larger growths. Micrometastases can generally be detected by routine histology. Some metastases are so small – only a few cells – that they require special staining techniques (immunohistochemistry) for their detection. The clinical significance of these tiny metastases is uncertain and still under investigation.

Despite the prognostic value of the number of involved lymph nodes, axillary dissection for nodal evaluation is on the wane. That technique is being replaced by sentinel lymph node examination. The change reflects an acknowledgment of the high degree of morbidity (that is, swelling of arm) associated with removal of the axillary lymph nodes.

The sentinel lymph node is the first node to drain the tumor. Hence, if that node is negative for tumor, the remaining lymph nodes are unlikely to harbor tumor. The reported accuracy of sentinel lymph node status in predicting axillary node status is approximately 96%.

If the sentinel lymph node is positive for tumor, axillary dissection is then usually carried out for both prognostic and therapeutic purposes.

Tumor size is an important factor in survival outcome. The larger the tumor, the greater the lymph node positivity. Size is also important independent of lymph node status. Among women with negative lymph nodes, the larger the size, the poorer the survival.

"Microinvasive" carcinomas are those in which the focus of invasion, in a setting of in situ carcinoma, measures no more than 1 mm. Patients with microinvasive carcinoma have a prognosis similar to that of patients with intraductal carcinoma alone.

Tumors larger than 1 mm but smaller than 5 mm are termed "minimal" carcinoma. Nevertheless, those tumors have the ability to metastasize and kill the patient.

Tumors 6 mm to 1 cm are still considered small. Breakpoints with respect to clinical staging occur at 5 mm, 1 cm, 2 cm, and 5 cm. The decision to administer chemotherapy is based in part on tumor size.

Tumor grade is another important factor with respect to prognosis. This factor is independent of tumor size and nodal status. The higher the grade, the shorter the survival.

Grading has already been discussed, but to reiterate briefly, the most commonly used grading system is based on three parameters: tumor architecture (tubule formation), nuclear grade, and mitotic activity. A scoring system incorporating these three parameters classifies tumors into grades 1, 2, and 3. The system is called modified Scarff–Bloom–Richardson. It is applicable chiefly to ordinary ductal carcinomas, but it can be applied to any tumor type.

Tumor type adds additional prognostic information, but is less important than grade. Carcinoma types other than ordinary infiltrating ductal carcinomas tend to have a better prognosis than that latter cancer. Many "good prognosis" tumor types are also grade 1. The relative significance of tumor types has already been discussed.

Flow cytometry is used to determine **DNA index (DNA ploidy)**. DNA index is often included in commercial laboratory panels for breast prognosis. Diploid tumors have a better prognosis, and aneuploid tumors have a worse prognosis. But ploidy tends to correlate with other prognostic factors; it may not be an independent prognostic factor.

The proliferative rate of a tumor is measured as **S-phase fraction**. The "fraction" reflects the percentage of tumor cells in the DNA synthesis phase of the cell cycle. It is measured by flow cytometry. A high S-phase fraction indicates faster growth and poorer overall survival. Mitotic activity, incorporated into tumor grade, is also a measure of proliferative rate. The S-phase fraction and tumor grade tend to run

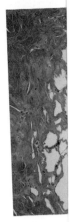

FIGURE 9.1

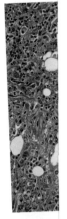

FIGURE 9

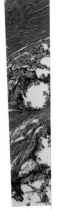

FIGURE

parallel to each other; they may not be independent of one another.

Potential prognostic indicators still under investigation include other oncogenes such as p53, enzymes that aid in invasiveness (such as cathepsin D), and measures of tumor angiogenesis such as microvessel density.

PREDICTIVE FACTORS

The **expression of estrogen receptors (ERs) and progesterone receptors (PRs)** is predictive of tumor response to hormone manipulation (tamoxifen). The correlation is imperfect, however. Approximately 77% of ER+PR+ tumors respond; approximately 27% of ER+PR– tumors respond; approximately 46% of ER–PR+ tumors respond; approximately 11% of ER–PR– tumors respond. Expression of estrogen and progesterone receptors is determined by immunohistochemical assay.

The gene **HER-2/*neu*** (cerbB2) codes for a protein, HER2, which is a cell membrane receptor that plays an important role in normal cell proliferation and differentiation. It comprises an extracellular binding component, a transmembrane component, and an intracellular component.

Activation of the extracellular portion by binding with the appropriate ligand leads to stimulation of the intracellular component, which sends signals to the nucleus to initiate cell division. When the HER2 protein is overexpressed – usually because of excess copies of the gene that codes for it, or because the protein becomes constitutively activated (that is, without the need for ligand binding) – cell division goes out of control (a feature of malignant transformation).

Overexpression of HER2 is a result of a genetic mutation. The abnormal gene is called an oncogene. Overexpression is determined by immunohistochemistry and HER-2/*neu* overamplification is determined by fluorescence in situ hybridization (FISH).

Overexpression of HER2 has generally indicated a more aggressive tumor with decreased responsiveness to tamoxifen and overall poorer prognosis. However, an antibody directed against HER2 has proven to be effective treatment against HER-2/*neu*–positive tumors. Overexpression of HER2 is now therefore considered to be a positive predictive indicator.

THE MALE BREAST

The most common lesion of the male breast is gynecomastia.

Carcinoma of the male breast is rare, but it does occur. The tumor types are similar to those that affect the female breast, the major differences being that infiltrating ductal carcinoma is relatively more common in men than in women (85% of breast carcinomas in men) and that infiltrating lobular carcinoma is exceptionally rare, presumably because lobules are not normally present in men. Estrogen and progesterone receptors are more often positive in men than in women. Often a tumor discovered in a man is more advanced owing to delay in diagnosis. However, the biology of breast carcinoma in men is very similar to that in women, and stage-for-stage, the prognosis is the same.

Figures 9.115 and 9.116

Gynecomastia is an enlargement of the breast that may be focal or diffuse, unilateral or bilateral. It is most often the result of drug therapy, but it may be idiopathic. It is characterized by a zone of periductal edema and inflammation, surrounded in turn by fibrosis (Figure 9.115). Typically, the ducts are hyper-

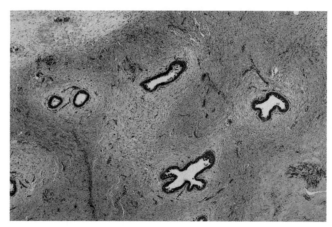

FIGURE 9.115

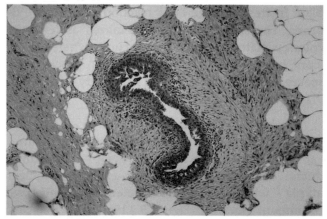

FIGURE 9.116

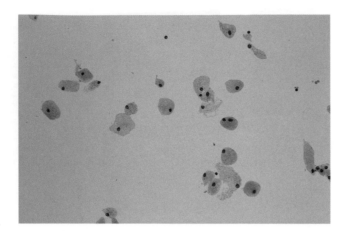

FIGURE 9.126

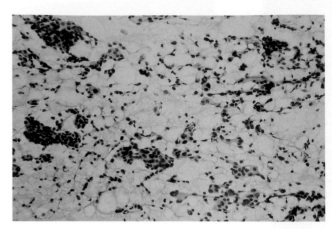

FIGURE 9.129

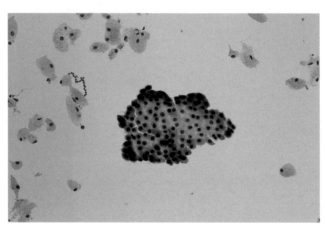

FIGURE 9.127

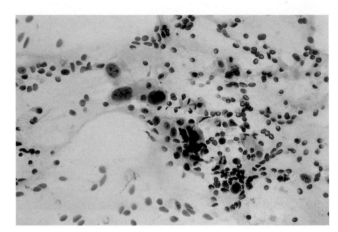

FIGURE 9.130

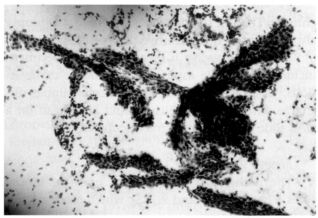

FIGURE 9.128

ing cells in branching stag horn–shaped configurations (Figure 9.128).

Figures 9.129 and 9.130
Carcinomas are characterized by smears that are highly cellular, with many single cells (Figure 9.129), and by cytologic atypia [nuclear enlargement, irregularity, and hyperchromasia (Figure 9.130)].

10

Role of the Surgeon— Biopsies

The role of the surgeon in a multidisciplinary approach to breast disease is unique because the surgeon interacts with the clinician, the radiologist, and the pathologist. Yet often, the surgeon is the first to see a patient with a breast problem.

Like any other physician, the surgeon must be aware of the incidences of the most common breast lesions and their clinical presentations. Using that information, he or she can determine the most appropriate surgical management. The surgeon should also know the limitations of mammography and should not rely simply on a negative mammogram in the presence of a palpable lesion.

Today's surgeon not only must know the relevant anatomy and possess the appropriate surgical skills, but must also be prepared to communicate with the radiologist and the pathologist. With the radiologist, the surgeon must be able to discuss mammography and ultrasound findings and guide-wire placement (in cases of imaging-guided needle biopsies). With the pathologist, the surgeon must seek to better understand the lesion so as to choose the most appropriate surgical treatment. (Seventy years ago, Bloodgood, a famous breast surgeon, said that the surgeon should also be his own pathologist. While that statement probably was true then, today it simply is not possible.)

The procedures that a surgeon has in the surgical armamentarium to diagnose and treat a breast lesion are

- fine-needle aspiration biopsy,
- core biopsy,
- incisional biopsy, and
- excisional biopsy.

FINE-NEEDLE ASPIRATION BIOPSY

Mammography and ultrasound examinations are never 100% accurate. The role of fine-needle aspiration biopsy (FNA) is to improve overall accuracy in assessing a breast lesion.

A cyst – especially when its fluid is under tension – may mimic a solid mass. In the case of a cyst, aspiration is not only diagnostic, but also therapeutic. If the cytology is negative, the cyst needs no further treatment.

An FNA procedure is simple and causes no trauma. It can be done in a physician's office. Local anesthesia is typically not required. (The needle used to administer a local agent would hurt as much as the aspiration.)

To obtain best cooperation from the patient and to ease fear of possible pain, the omission of anesthesia must be explained before the procedure. The discomfort of the procedure can be described as being equal to a venipuncture or vaccination.

INDICATIONS
An FNA is indicated for

- pathology analysis of any palpable lesion of the breast – whether mass or tumor, discrete nodule, or ill-defined breast-tissue thickening.
- determination of whether a mass is cystic or solid.
- pathology analysis for patients with a history of fibrocystic mastopathy manifested with a dominant mass in the breast that does not disappear with the menstrual cycle.
- preoperative diagnosis. If the pathology report notes malignant cells, the surgical treatment can be discussed preoperatively with the patient. It must be emphasized, however, that final treatment should never be formulated from an FNA diagnosis alone. Cytopathology findings from a core biopsy, a frozen section, or a permanent section should be used to confirm the diagnosis.

- determination of whether a large cancer should be downstaged with chemotherapy before a mastectomy.
- confirmation of a suspected locally recurrent carcinoma after lumpectomy or mastectomy.
- confirmation of a clinical diagnosis in a pregnant woman in her first trimester. If an FNA confirms a clinical diagnosis of a benign lesion, then the excision can be postponed until later in the pregnancy or after delivery.

PROCEDURE

The aspiration can be done with the patient in the upright or supine position. The author prefers the patient to be supine, because that position is more comfortable for the patient and because the physician can steady the lesion against the chest wall more efficiently. To better facilitate the procedure in patients who have pendulous breasts or whose lesion is near the axilla or in the lower quadrants of the breast, the patient should elevate the ipsilateral arm overhead.

Figure 10.1

Only a few tools and supplies are necessary for performing an FNA:

- Syringe, 10 mL
- Alcohol swab
- Needle, clear plastic, 22 gauge, 1.5 inches long
- Dry gauze, 2 in. × 2 in.
- Glass slides

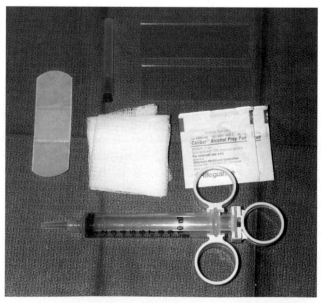

FIGURE 10.1

Figure 10.2

The skin is cleansed with the alcohol swab. The mass is then secured and steadied by being grasped between the thumb and index finger of the physician's non-dominant hand. The plunger of the syringe should be at the zero mark when the needle is inserted into the breast.

In the case of a cyst, the needle "falls in." The fluid is then aspirated. A complete collapse of the cyst can be accomplished by pressing the supporting fingers down against the cyst.

If the mass is solid and can be penetrated, some amount of tissue can almost always be aspirated. A simple way to know that the needle is indeed in the lesion is to use the supporting fingers to move the lesion. The needle will oscillate if it is in the correct location. If the mass is malignant, a "gritty" sensation is felt, comparable to piercing an apple or a potato.

With the needle in good position, the physician creates suction in the syringe by pulling the plunger toward the 10 mL mark. At the same time, the physician moves the needle backward and forward in one plane until some material appears in the needle hub.

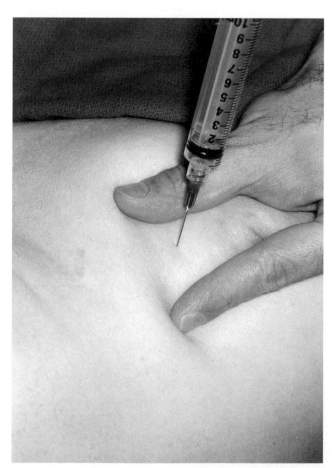

FIGURE 10.2

To obtain a good sample, two or three passes in various directions are recommended.

When sufficient material has been obtained, the physician releases the plunger and only then withdraws the needle. This sequence prevents material from being sucked into the syringe.

Pressure is applied at the site of the aspiration for a few minutes.

For lesions located behind the nipple–areola complex, the physician should insert the needle laterally from outside the areola margin, because piercing the areola skin is more painful than piercing the adjacent skin.

Figure 10.3

When the lesion is located in a medial quadrant, the physician should stand on the side opposite to the quadrant where the lesion is located.

In Figure 10.3, an FNA being done on the patient's right breast. The patient is turned slightly in a medial decubitus toward the side where the procedure is taking place. The lesion can then be entered tangentially, with the needle running almost parallel to the chest wall, avoiding the possibility of a pneumothorax.

Figure 10.4

To transfer all the material lodged in the needle hub, the needle should be detached from the syringe and then filled with air.

Figures 10.5 and 10.6

The needle is reattached to the air-filled syringe, and the material is squirted onto a glass slide. Steadying the first slide with one hand, the physician

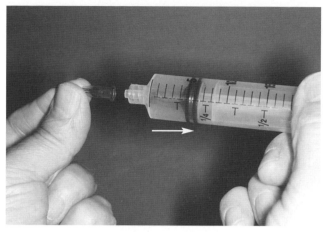

FIGURE 10.4

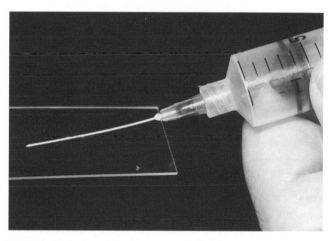

FIGURE 10.5

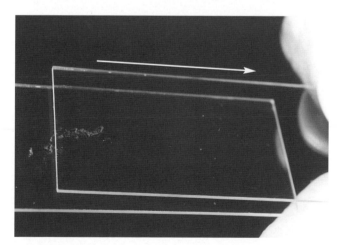

FIGURE 10.6

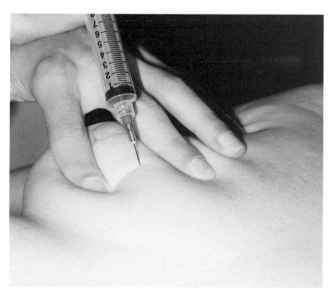

FIGURE 10.3

creates a smear of the extracted material by sliding the material with another slide glass.

At least two (preferably three) passes should be made, with the resulting smears separately labeled. Preparation of the smears depends on preference of

the cytopathologist. Before sending specimens, the physician should always consult with that professional regarding the preferred technique.

If the cytology is not revealing, a repeat physical examination, mammogram, or aspiration should be recommended within two to three months. (Ultrasound and stereotactic guided core biopsy are discussed in chapter 8, "Role of the Radiologist.")

COMPLICATIONS

Aside from minor ecchymosis and hematoma, a carefully done FNA should cause no complications. Careful sterile technique should prevent infection. Pneumothorax is unusual, but it is nevertheless a possibility in cases where the lesion is posterior and near the chest wall.

CORE BIOPSY

Another tool available to the surgeon is a Mammotome® core biopsy device. A larger amount of tissue can be obtained using that instrument.

A Mammotome core biopsy can be an office procedure. It requires only a few drops of a local anesthetic and a small incision for introduction of the needle.

The procedure is restricted to palpable tumors that have been diagnosed using ultrasonography or mammography and that are not deeply seated within the breast. The procedure is carried out by the radiologist. (See chapter 8, "Role of the Radiologist.")

The most common complication of the procedure is (usually controllable) bleeding.

INCISIONAL BIOPSY

Incisional biopsy is reserved for large tumors and for confirming clinical suspicion of an inflammatory carcinoma so that chemotherapy can be used to downstage the disease before a definitive procedure. (See chapter 12, Figures 2.34 and 2.35, for the surgical procedure.) (For The Surgical Procedure, see chapter 2 Figures 2.34 and 2.35.)

EXCISIONAL BIOPSY

A breast excisional biopsy is also called lumpectomy. It is the complete removal of a well-defined mass or tumor.

Excisional biopsy is indicated for situations in which

- an FNA fails to produce a diagnosis, and
- a diagnosis of carcinoma is made using ultrasound-guided or stereotactic-guided core biopsy.

Before definitive surgical and adjuvant treatment is determined, a lumpectomy alone is nowadays almost a standard initial treatment for breast cancer.

11

Surgical Treatment of Benign Breast Lesions

Most breast lesions are benign and the most commonly excised benign breast tumors are fibroadenomas.

EXCISION OF A SINGLE BENIGN TUMOR

Fibroadenomas are well encapsulated lesions (see chapter 1, "Benign Tumors," Figure 1.10). They can be excised by enucleating them from the surrounding breast tissue.

In young patients, fibroadenomas may be excised without including a rim of normal-appearing breast tissue surrounding the capsule. In older patients, especially as they approach the age at which the incidence of breast cancer peaks, the excision should include such a rim. See "Surgical Technique – Lumpectomy" later in this chapter. Here, the excision of a single benign breast tumor is discussed.

Surgical Technique – Single Fibroadenoma

The procedure is typically done in an outpatient facility. Local anesthesia and monitored intravenous sedation are used.

PREPARATION AND ANESTHESIA

Figure 11.1
The patient is positioned eccentrically on the operating table, with the side being operated on near the edge of the table. For patients who have pendulous breasts, or whose lesion is located in a lateral quadrant of the breast, a pad placed under the ipsilateral side of the chest may help with breast positioning.

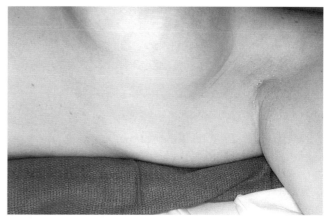

FIGURE 11.1

Figures 11.2 and 11.3
The local anesthetic agent is injected into two separate planes: the subcutaneous tissue layer (Figure 11.2) and the breast parenchyma. If the lesion is located deep within the breast, the local anesthetic is also injected deep to the lesion. The needle is introduced below and behind the lesion, just above the breast crease and parallel to the chest wall. The anesthetic agent is injected as the needle is withdrawn (Figure 11.3).

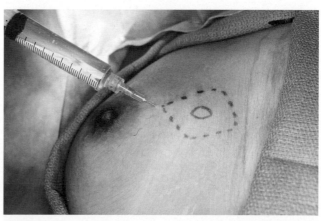

FIGURE 11.2

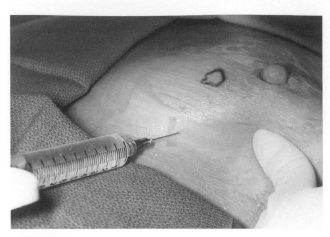

FIGURE 11.3

INCISION

Figure 11.4

Except in the case of lesions located near or behind the areola (for which a curvilinear circumareolar incision is the incision of choice), a radial incision should be made over the area where the tumor is located. The incision should be large enough to facilitate good exposure.

To avoid or minimize a hypertrophic scar, radial incisions should follow the Kraissl's skin lines. Unlike the Langer's skin lines, which were described in the cadaver, Kraissl's lines are the dynamic lines of the skin, which run perpendicular to the direction of the

underlying muscle fibers. Because the pectoralis muscle fibers run in an oblique direction from their origin at their clavicular, sternal, and abdominal insertions to their insertion at the humerus, a radial incision can be made in nearly every quadrant of the breast.

Figure 11.4 shows a radial incision in the upper outer quadrant of the right breast for excision of a fibroadenoma located near the tail of Spence.

Figures 11.5 and 11.6

When the lesion is superficial and close to the areolar margin, incisions along the areolar skin margin are ideal (Figures 11.5 and 11.6). For tumors located near the edge of the areola but away from the margin, a circumareolar incision can also be used. As shown in Figure 11.6, an incision was extended halfway around the circumference of the areola. The skin flap was dissected to pass the area of the tumor, providing good exposure and access to the tumor. Tunneling through the breast should be avoided, especially if cancer is suspected.

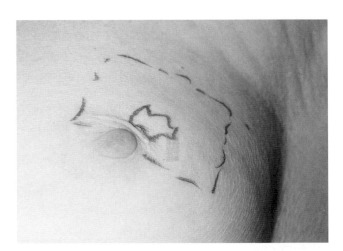

FIGURE 11.5

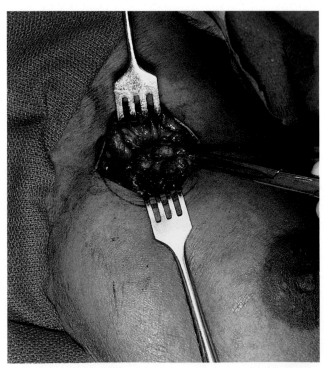

FIGURE 11.4

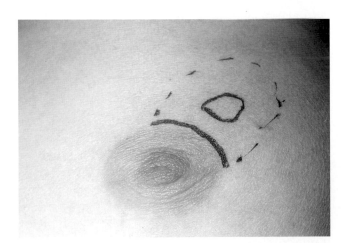

FIGURE 11.6

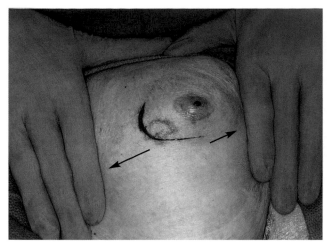

FIGURE 11.7

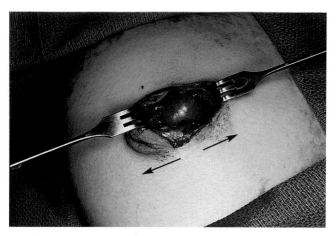

FIGURE 11.8

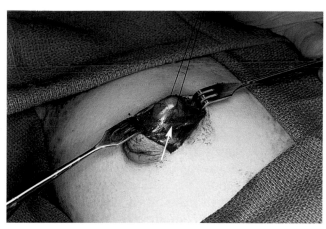

FIGURE 11.9

Figure 11.7

The areola skin may be wrinkled and its edge irregular. This appearance is more common in multiparous patients and in patients with pendulous breasts. To obtain a straight, even circumareolar incision in such cases, the skin should be stretched down and out as shown in Figure 11.7 (arrows).

Figure 11.8

The skin incision is deepened through the subcutaneous tissue to the breast tissue layer. That layer is easy to recognize because of its whitish color, which contrasts with the yellow color of the subcutaneous tissue. Hemostasis is achieved using electrocautery.

Two skin flaps (including skin and subcutaneous tissue) are raised by sharp dissection and extended far enough to provide good exposure (arrows).

EXCISION

Figure 11.9

Fibroadenomas are separated from the surrounding breast tissue by a layer of fibrous connective tissue (arrow). They can be excised by sharp dissection in that cleavage-tissue plane. Dissecting scissors can be used. Excision can be facilitated by placing traction on the lesion as the dissection progresses. If, at any point in the dissection, the lesion appears indeterminate, then it should be removed with a rim of normal breast tissue so that the margins can be studied.

Figure 11.10

Dissection of the lesion continues around its circumference until only the vascular pedicle is keeping the lesion attached to the capsule. The pedicle carries the blood supply. It should be clamped and tied before transection.

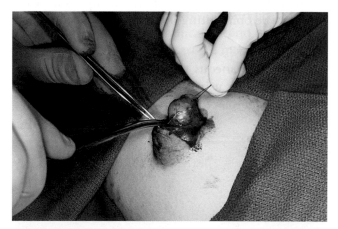

FIGURE 11.10

CLOSURE

Figure 11.11

To obtain a good cosmetic result and to minimize a hypertrophic scar or keloid, the defect in the breast should be carefully approximated in its

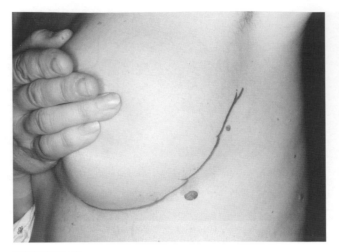

FIGURE 11.18

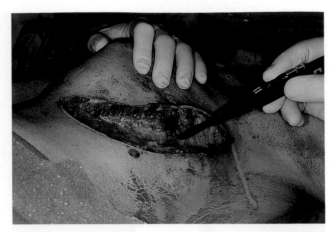

FIGURE 11.20

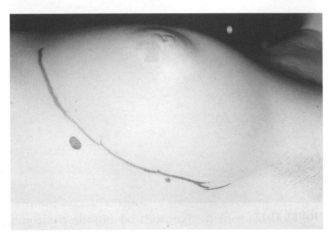

FIGURE 11.19

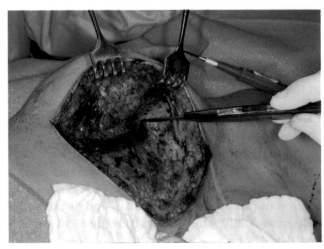

FIGURE 11.21

Figure 11.19

A small pillow placed beneath the patient's back on the ipsilateral side of the lesion elevates the latissimus dorsi muscle. The skin is cleansed with an antiseptic solution.

INCISION

Figure 11.20

The incision commences approximately 3–4 cm below the axilla. It follows the breast crease and curves medially toward the sternum, extending laterally toward the sternum approximately 3–4 cm.

Figure 11.21

The incision is deepened through the subcutaneous tissue until the serratus anterior and the pectoralis major muscles are exposed.

EXCISION

Figure 11.22

The dissection is now carried medially along the retromammary space between the posterior surface of the breast and the deep layer of the pectoralis fascia. This space is largely avascular. Small bleeders have to be cauterized only occasionally. The dissection continues medially until the lateral border of the sternum is reached. This ample dissection allows the breast to be completely freed from the chest wall and inverted. The surgeon accomplishes the inversion by placing the non-dominant hand into the retromammary space and by pushing the breast with the dominant hand.

Figure 11.23

With the posterior surface of the breast exposed, each tumor is manually localized and individually pushed toward the exposed posterior surface of the

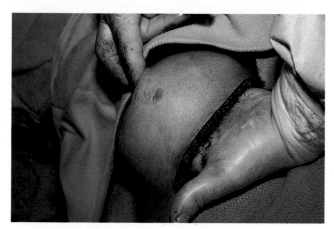

FIGURE 11.22

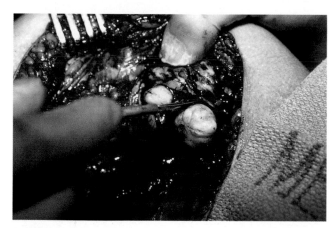

FIGURE 11.23

breast. The breast parenchyma overlying each tumor is incised. Once the tumor is exposed, it is shelled out of its capsule. All the tumors are excised using the same technique.

CLOSURE

When hemostasis is complete, each rent in the breast tissue is individually closed with 2/0 chromic catgut sutures. The wound is irrigated with lukewarm water to uncover any open bleeding vessels that remain. The breast is then returned to its place.

A drain that will be connected to a constant negative-pressure device is placed between the chest wall and the posterior surface of the breast. This drain remains in place until drainage is negligible.

The subcutaneous tissue is closed with 2/0 plain catgut, and the skin with a subcuticular stitch using absorbable monofilament suture. A pressure dressing is applied to the chest wall.

The synchronous, bilateral, multiple fibroadenomas excised from this patient's breasts are shown in chapter 1, "Benign Tumors," Figure 1.11 and Figure

1.12. The patient had ten fibroadenomas on the right breast and eight on the left breast. The surgical procedures were staged as two separate interventions.

Figure 11.24
Figure 11.24 shows the patient's postoperative appearance (arms raised). When the patient's arms are by her side, the scar is hidden in the breast crease.

Surgical Technique – Large Phyllodes Tumor

Phyllodes tumors are more common in older patients (who are approaching the age at which the incidence of breast cancer peaks). Patients with a clinical suspected phyllodes tumor should therefore have a core biopsy before any surgical procedure. The core biopsy will provide a definitive histopathology assessment that assists in planning the surgical management.

PREPARATION, INCISION, AND DISSECTION
The preoperative preparation, incision, and dissection of the breast from the pectoralis major muscle proceed as described for multiple fibroadenomas (preceding subsection). Also, the retromammary space is dissected and the breast is everted as described previously.

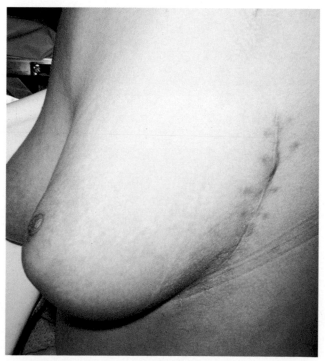

FIGURE 11.24

EXCISION

Figures 11.25 and 11.26

To prevent a local recurrence, the excision of a phyllodes tumor must include a rim of normal breast tissue approximately 1–2 cm in width. (The clinical presentation of the tumor being excised here is shown in chapter 1, "Benign Tumors," Figure 1.34.)

Figure 11.27

To facilitate the excision and to avoid injury to the skin or the nipple, the assistant surgeon should, as he is applying upward traction to the breast, "push" the outer surface of the breast with the forefingers as shown in Figure 11.27.

Figure 11.28

The patient in Figure 11.28 was treated surgically for a large phyllodes tumor. The nipple is retracted because the dissection closely approached the nipple, causing the loss of symmetry.

When a resection is treating a large tumor and the defect in the breast is considerable, an augmen-

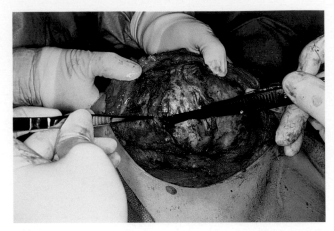

FIGURE 11.27

tation mammoplasty may be necessary. This reconstructive procedure should be delayed until the histopathology of the tumor is known.

CLOSURE

Closure also proceeds as described for multiple fibroadenomas. The wound is drained with a negative-pressure suction device.

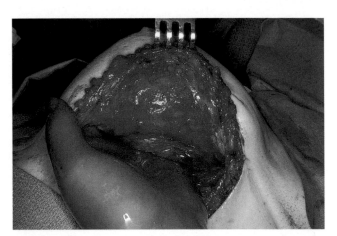

FIGURE 11.25

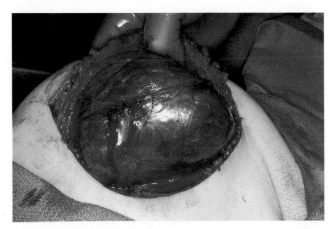

FIGURE 11.26

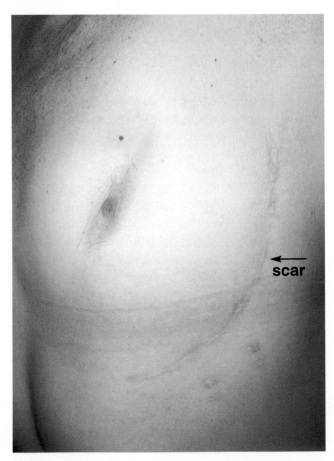

scar

FIGURE 11.28

COMPLICATIONS

Major complications are almost entirely absent with this procedure.

The patient should be restricted from vigorous arm and shoulder exercise for two to three weeks after surgery so that the breast has time to form enough fibrous tissue to re-adhere to the chest wall.

EXCISION OF THE MAJOR DUCTS OF THE BREAST

The major ducts of the breast are the milk ducts located directly behind the areola. Milk is conducted to the nipple through 15–20 main ducts (called "lobular ducts"). Before each lobular duct reaches the nipple, it dilates, forming a ductal sinus (see Figure 11.34).

Distal to the sinus, the ducts continue to converge into ducts called the major ducts, each of which takes the shape of an inverted bottle neck. Two or more sinuses may converge into one major duct. Approximately 8–10 major ducts are located in the retroareolar area. Each one surfaces at a separate nipple orifice.

Indications for an excision of the major ducts of the breast are

- spontaneous serous, serosanguineous, bloody, or watery discharge (Figure 11.29);
- chronic retroareolar abscesses (Figure 11.30);
- chronic, recurrent infections of the periareolar area (Figure 11.31);
- intractable chronic, recurrent infections of the periareolar area (Figure 11.32); and
- failure to remove an underlying pathology when only the "affected duct" was excised (Figure 11.33).

The procedure is contraindicated in women under the age of 30 and in older women who are anxious to have children and nurse. In those patients an attempt should be made to single out and excise the affected duct.

Figure 11.29

The patient in Figure 11.29 was treated surgically for a spontaneous bloody discharge from the right nipple. A soft tumor was palpable at the 11 o'clock position on the right breast near the areola. It measured approximately 1 cm in diameter. Finger pressure on the area of the tumor produced a bloody discharge.

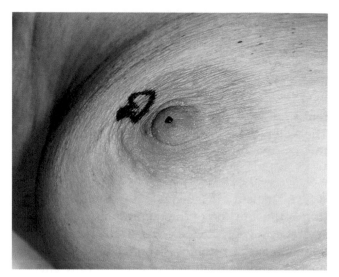

FIGURE 11.29

Although serous, serosanguineous, and bloody nipple discharge are caused by microscopic intraductal papillomas, a combination of macroscopic and microscopic papillomas is not infrequent.

Excision of the major ducts and the tumor resolved the problem.

Figure 11.30

The patient in Figure 11.30 had a chronic retroareolar abscess with spontaneous drainage through the nipple. The acute symptoms of fever and pain subsided each time the drainage occurred. Because of the chronic nature of the symptom, an excision of the central ducts was performed in the chronic phase of

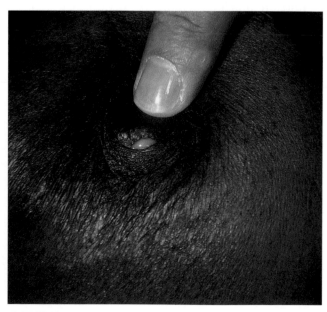

FIGURE 11.30

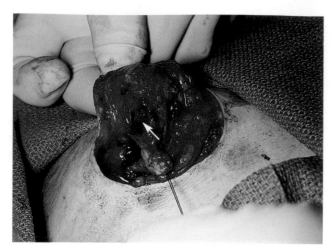

FIGURE 11.38

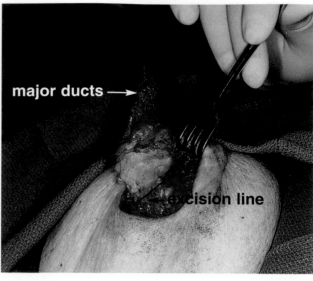

FIGURE 11.40

index finger of the non-dominant hand to push the nipple inward as transection of the ducts proceeds.

Figure 11.39

Occasionally aberrant extra ducts are found (arrow). The aberrant duct in Figure 11.39 was connected to an independent nipple orifice. When such ducts harbor pathology, they may be dilated with dark or blue-colored fluid. They should also be excised.

Figure 11.40

The line of excision takes a quadrangular rotated-diamond shape with the deepening of the incision about 1–2 cm down into the breast tissue. The

major ducts and some of the surrounding breast tissue are removed. The diamond shaped excision facilitates the cosmetic closure of the rent, maintaining the shape and contour of the breast postoperatively.

Figure 11.41

A bisected specimen demonstrates the multicentricity of the lesion. Blood is prasent in multiple ducts.

Because papillomas are usually microscopic and soft, a frozen section is not done. Rather, the entire specimen is submitted for permanent paraffin sections. The suture used to tie the major ducts before the transection and an additional suture placed on the lateral margin will assist the pathologist in situating the specimen.

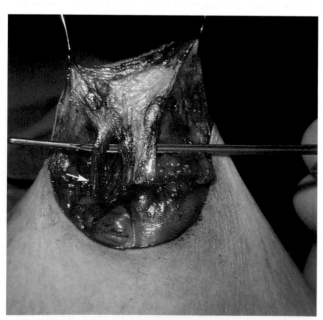

FIGURE 11.39

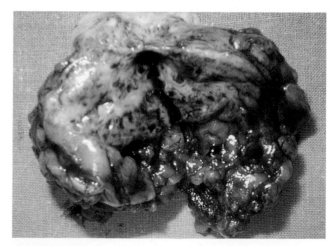

FIGURE 11.41

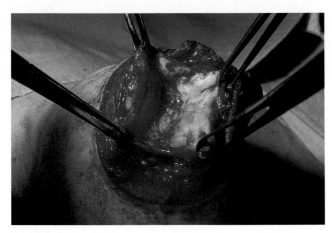

FIGURE 11.42

Figure 11.42

After hemostasis is achieved, the cut surface of the breast should be expressed and searched for seepage of fluid though the transected ducts. Fluid issuing through the cut surface of the ducts indicates that additional pathology still exists distal to the resection. Further excision should be done until no more fluid is observed. Figure 11.42 shows the rent in the breast tissue resulting from the excision of the central ducts.

CLOSURE

Figure 11.43

After hemostasis has been achieved and the wound irrigated, the incision can be closed. Closure of the breast tissue occurs in layers. The breast tissue layer is approximated using 2/0 chromic catgut sutures. The subcutaneous tissue is closed in line using 3/0 plain catgut sutures. The skin layer is closed

using a continuous subcuticular stitch and 4/0 monofilament absorbable suture.

Figure 11.44A and 11.44B

Figure 11.44 shows the nipple–areola complex at the end of the surgical procedure (A). A drain is usually unnecessary, because the nipple orifices serve as drainage openings. A pressure dressing with a cutout at the center of the gauze (B) will assist the drainage and also prevent flattening of the nipple.

Figure 11.45

The patient in Figure 11.45 had the major ducts excised from the right breast. Postoperatively, no loss of breast contour or change in the shape or appearance of the nipple is seen.

COMPLICATIONS

Occasionally, a seroma may collect under the areola. A needle aspiration will resolve the complication.

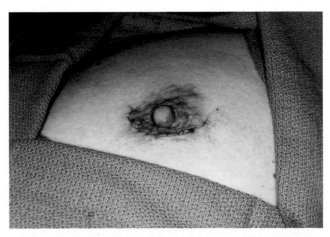

FIGURE 11.44A

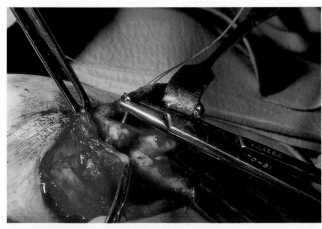

FIGURE 11.43

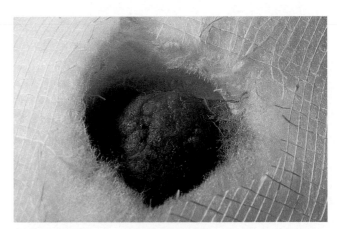

FIGURE 11.44B

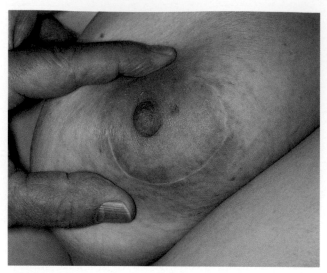

FIGURE 11.45

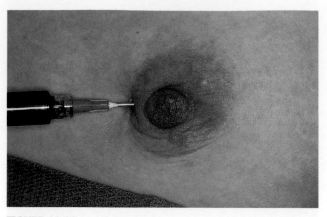

FIGURE 11.46

SURGICAL TREATMENT OF CHRONIC, RECURRENT PERIAREOLAR INFECTION

Chronic periareolar or retroareolar abscesses are usually connected to the major duct system of the breast by a fistulous tract (see Figure 11.32). To resolve the problem, the fistula should be excised in continuity with the major ducts.

Surgical Technique – Periareolar Infection

As with an excision of the major ducts alone, an excision of the major ducts and fistulae can be performed in an ambulatory setting under local infiltrative anesthesia and monitored intravenous sedation.

PREPARATION

Figure 11.46

After skin preparation and draping, methylene blue is instilled into the fistula tract. A 20-gauge blunt needle is usually adequate. Instillation of the dye should be slow and gentle to prevent extravasation.

INCISION

Figure 11.47

A circumareolar incision is made. The incision should extend for 180 degrees along the inferior areola circumference. It should include a portion of the skin that contains the external fistula opening. The areola skin is elevated as described for simple excision of the major ducts (see Figures 11.35 and 11.36).

EXCISION

Figure 11.48

The fistula tract is dissected off the skin and underlying breast tissue. It will be incorporated into the specimen. A skin hook is used to hold the skin containing the fistula opening in traction while dissection of the areola skin flap is completed.

Figure 11.49

The breast tissue containing the central ducts and the fistulous tract is excised in a rotated-dia-

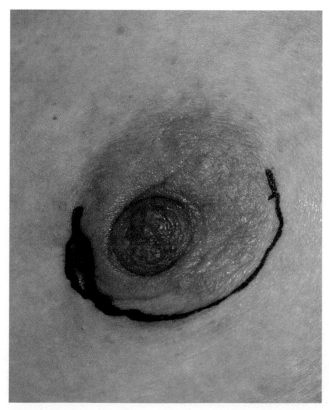

FIGURE 11.47

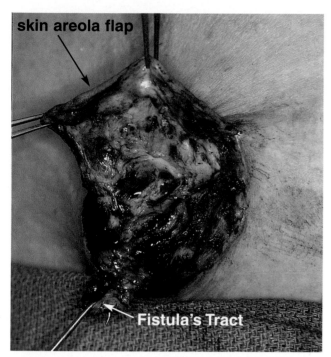

FIGURE 11.48

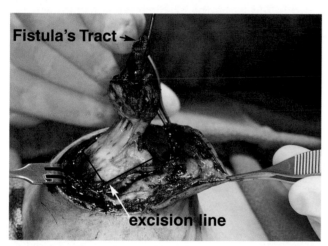

FIGURE 11.49

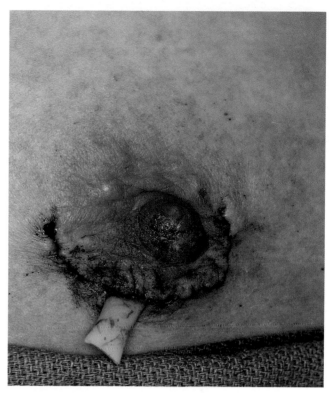

FIGURE 11.50

mond shape to facilitate the cosmetic closure of the breast parenchyma. The excision should be wide enough to insure complete removal of the affected tissues.

Dye in the operative field during the dissection indicates that pathology still exists distal to the excised area. The excision should be widened until non-stained breast tissue is encountered.

CLOSURE

Figure 11.50

The wound is closed with non-absorbable interrupted sutures. Because of this procedure's potential for infection, the wound should always be drained. The drain should remain in place for two to three days. The pressure dressing should have a cutout that accommodates the nipple and prevents its collapse [see Figure 11.44(B)].

IMAGING-GUIDED BIOPSY

With the increased use of screening mammography, small breast lesions are now being detected before they become palpable. Effective excision of such lesions requires the combined efforts of the radiologist and the surgeon.

The localization procedure for nonpalpable lesions was discussed in chapter 8, "Role of the Radiologist." The surgical technique for excising such lesions is discussed here.

The indications for imaging-guided excisions are

- discovery of small nonpalpable breast tumors with a stellate configuration,
- discovery of a new cluster of heterogeneous calcifications of an indeterminate type,
- return of positive cytology results from an ultrasound-guided or stereotactic-guided core biopsy on any breast lesion,

- technical impossibility of performing a stereotactic-guided biopsy, and
- increase in the size of a solid nonpalpable mass that images as benign.

The excision of tumors that image mammographically as strictly benign should be left to the judgment of the surgeon. That professional should make the decision based on the patient's risk factors for breast carcinoma and her degree of anxiety.

Surgical Technique – Imaging-Guided Biopsy

An imaging-guided biopsy is done in an ambulatory facility under local anesthesia and monitored intravenous sedation.

PREPARATION

On the day of the scheduled procedure, the Radiology department localizes the lesion as described in chapter 8, "Role of the Radiologist." The guide wire

is placed at, or as close as possible to the lesion, and final mediolateral oblique (MLO) and cephalic-caudal (CC) mammogram views are obtained.

Figure 11.51A and 11.51B

The surgeon and the radiologist should discuss the post-localization mammograms and, together, fix the coordinates that determine the exact location of the wire in relation to the lesion (A). The distance from the lesion to the skin is also measured (B). The nipple is the point of reference.

Figures 11.52 and 11.53

The local anesthetic is injected into the subcutaneous tissue and the breast tissue adjacent to the lesion (A). If the lesion is located posterior in the breast, local anesthetic should also be injected in a plane posterior to the lesion (B). To inject local anesthetic into the tissue posterior to the lesion, the breast is retracted cephalad to expose the crease, Figure 11.53 (arrow). The needle enters just above the crease and is introduced past the lesion, parallel to the chest wall (B). The anesthetic agent is injected as the needle is being withdrawn.

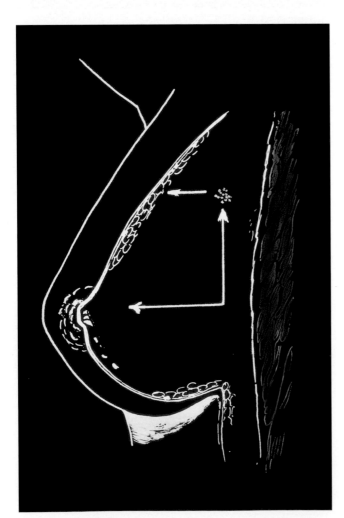

FIGURE 11.51A

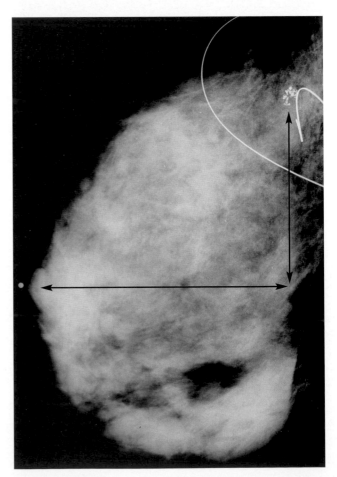

FIGURE 11.51B

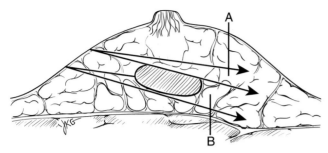

FIGURE 11.52

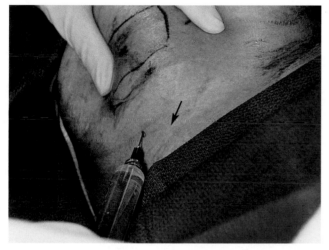

FIGURE 11.53

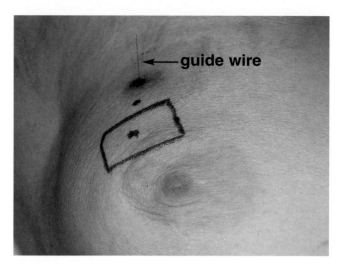

FIGURE 11.54

Figure 11.54

The approximate location of the lesion and the extent of the excision are mapped using the coordinates fixed from the post-localization mammogram. The estimated area of excision is also mapped.

INCISION

The guide wire is trimmed where it protrudes through the patient's skin, leaving a stub approximately 2–3 cm long outside the breast. Because the wire is potentially contaminated and because it will be retrieved into the operative field at a certain point in the procedure, prophylactic intravenous antibiotics should be administered at the start of surgery.

The breast skin and the protruding wire stub are cleansed with a skin preparation solution. The arm and the entire breast from the clavicle to the upper abdomen are prepped. The operating table may be tilted away from or toward the surgeon depending on the quadrant in which the lesion is located.

The skin incision is made at the coordinates that mark the location of the lesion. If the lesion is close to the areola, a circumareolar incision is preferable. Radial incisions should follow the Kraissl's skin lines. Those skin lines run perpendicular to the fibers of the underlying muscle. Because the muscle fibers of the pectoralis major muscle run almost vertically from the abdomen to the clavicle and the humerus, the skin lines of the breast are almost always on a radial axis. The incision is also planned so that it can accommodate more radical surgery should such surgery be indicated.

Figure 11.55

Whether the localizing wire enters the breast on the perpendicular or at an angle (Figure 11.55), the author prefers to make the skin incision at the site of the lesion (X) and not where the needle enters the skin. In the author's experience, a second incision to retrieve the wire is seldom necessary.

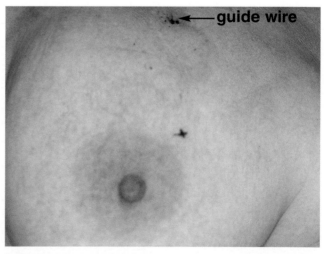

FIGURE 11.55

Figure 11.56

The incision is deepened through the subcutaneous tissue down to the breast parenchyma. (The breast parenchyma is recognizable because of its whitish color, which contrasts with the yellow color of the subcutaneous tissue.) On the plane between the subcutaneous layer and the parenchyma two skin flaps are raised and extended to the estimated line of resection.

Figure 11.57

Once the skin flaps are complete, the localizing wire is retrieved into the operative field. The dissection is carried in a plane between the subcutaneous tissue and the breast parenchyma by serially opening and closing the clamp or scissors as the dissection progresses toward the wire. The wire's point of entry into the breast can be estimated by putting gentle traction on the external portion of the wire as the dissection progresses.

Figure 11.58

Upon reaching the wire, the surgeon uses a clamp to grasp it and retrieve it into the operative field.

EXCISION

Figure 11.59

Once the wire has been retrieved into the operative field, the segment of the breast containing the

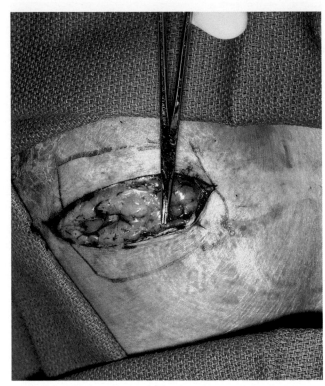

FIGURE 11.58

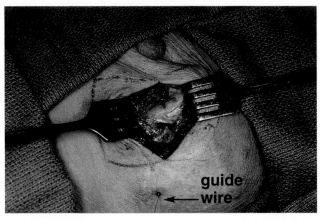

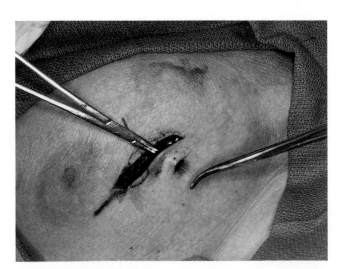

FIGURE 11.56

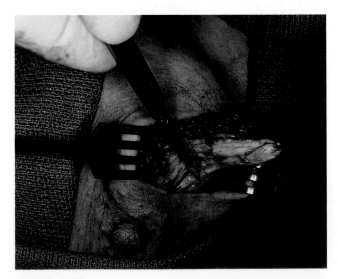

FIGURE 11.57   FIGURE 11.59

lesion and the localizing wire is placed in traction. Either an Allis clamp or a silk suture can be used. The author prefers the suture, as that method prevents trauma to the tissue that may create a problem during the histopathology interpretation.

A wide segment of breast parenchyma is resected to achieve tumor-free margins. The excision should be accomplished by sharp dissection with a scalpel (avoid dissecting scissors). Using the scalpel avoids leaving serrated edges whose crevices may hide capillary oozing. The result for the breast parenchyma is better healing without distortion.

As the excision progresses, the surgeon should continually check the wire to prevent its accidental transection.

If the lesion is malignant and if adequate margins were obtained, the biopsy procedure may serve as the lumpectomy portion of a breast-conserving treatment.

Figure 11.60

A specimen mammogram is obtained to check that the lesion was completely excised and that the localizing wire is intact.

Figure 11.61

For margin evaluation, sutures should be used to situate the specimen. Two sutures are sufficient: a short suture for the superior margin (short = superior) and a long suture for the lateral margin (long = lateral). Accurate situation and inking of the specimen surface can help in the determination of whether the margins are free or which (if any) are positive. Consistency of labeling prevents errors in communication with the pathologist.

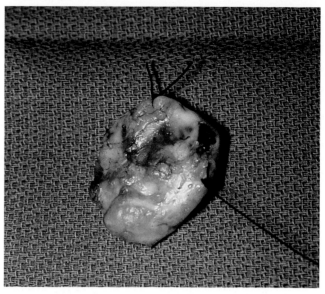

FIGURE 11.61

The wound should be inspected for residual areas of thickening. Any indurated or suspicious areas should also be excised. The margins of subsequent specimens should be situated in the same manner as the first.

Figures 11.62 and 11.63

Multiple small lesions or multifocal clusters of microcalcifications may require the localization of each individual lesion. Lesions that are sufficiently close to one another can all be excised with only one incision. Otherwise, multiple incisions may be required.

CLOSURE

The wound closure proceeds in layers as described for excision of a single fibroadenoma (see Figures 11.11 through 11.17).

The rent in the breast tissue created by the excision of the lesion is closed with 2/0 chromic catgut using interrupted stitches. Depending on the size of the rent, more than one layer of stitches may be necessary.

The skin flaps are approximated by first suturing the subcutaneous tissue with interrupted sutures using 2/0 plain catgut. To prevent tension at the suture line, the dermal layer is also approximated. Sutures of 3/0 plain catgut are used.

The skin is approximated using continuous sutures of absorbable monofilament material placed in the subcuticular layer of the skin.

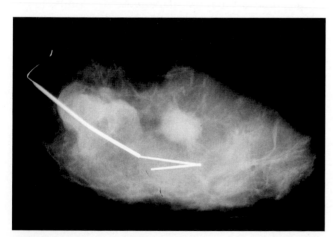

FIGURE 11.60

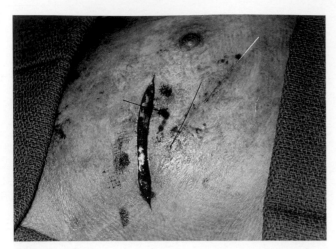

FIGURE 11.62

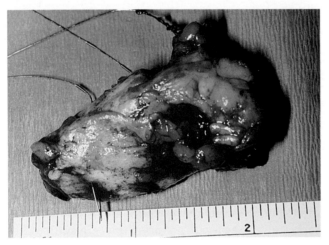

FIGURE 11.63

EXCISION OF GYNECOMASTIA

The indications for surgery in cases of gynecomastia are essentially cosmetic and psychological. Gynecomastias are occasionally symptomatic; but, with reassurance, surgery may be avoided. Gynecomastia in the pubertal age is physiologic. In these patients, surgery should be postponed for two to three years after the diagnosis, during which time the gynecomastia may resolve spontaneously.

Where fat is chiefly responsible for the enlargement of the breast (lipomastia), liposuction rather than surgery may be an adequate treatment. If the lipomastia is accompanied by a firm glandular component (an associated gynecomastia), the condition should be treated surgically.

Surgical Technique – Gynecomastia

Excision of a gynecomastia is the male equivalent of a female total mastectomy. The excision is performed through a periareolar incision. This relatively simple surgical procedure carries minimal morbidity.

The surgery can be done in an outpatient facility. Small gynecomastias can be excised under local anesthesia and monitored intravenous sedation. For very large gynecomastias, general anesthesia is recommended.

PREPARATION AND ANESTHESIA

With the patient positioned on the operating table, the skin of the affected breast is prepared with an antiseptic solution.

The local anesthetic agent should be infiltrated superficially and deep to the gynecomastia (see Figure 11.52). To infiltrate the retromammary space, the surgeon should grasp the breast between the fingers and the thumb and lift the breast. The needle enters just above the breast crease and is advanced parallel to the chest wall. The anesthetic agent is injected as the needle is being withdrawn.

INCISION

Figures 11.64 and 11.65
Because the blood supply to the nipple–areola complex comes from the superior quadrants, the incision is made in the circumareolar line, along the inferior margin (Figure 11.64). This incision also makes the dissection technically more comfortable for the surgeon.

An incision extending for a hemi-circumference (180 degrees) is usually adequate for excising small gynecomastias. For larger gynecomastias, a circumareolar incision may be inadequate for complete excision of the gland. In such cases, transverse radial extensions are made on the 3 o'clock and 9 o'clock radii (Figure 11.65).

Figure 11.66
The incision is now deepened into the gynecomastia for 5–10 mm, leaving a rim of breast tissue under the areola skin flap. In that cleavage plane, the flap is completed. Leaving this small portion of the gland attached under the areola (A) and preserving some of the retromammary fat (B) minimizes postoperative deformity. This cleavage plane is extended by sharp dissection parallel to the overlying skin.

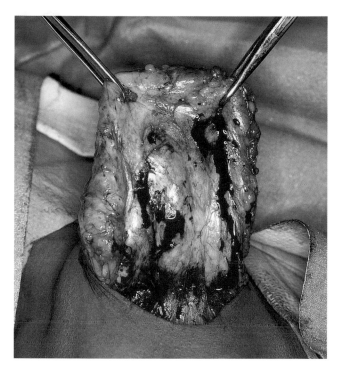

FIGURE 11.64

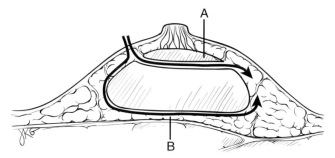

FIGURE 11.66

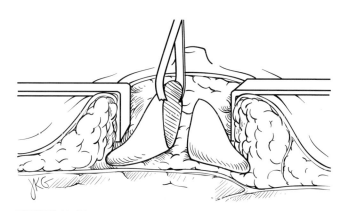

FIGURE 11.67

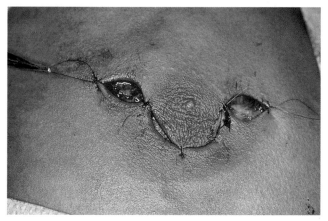

FIGURE 11.65

EXCISION

Figure 11.67

When the gynecomastia is large and even the radial extensions are inadequate to permit the excision of the entire gland, the gynecomastia should be bisected. The bisection is accomplished by cutting perpendicularly through the gland to the thoracic wall. After the breast has been bisected, each half is removed separately.

CLOSURE

Once hemostasis is complete, the wound is irrigated with sterile water to remove any remaining blood clots that may be hiding open capillaries or small blood vessels.

The excision of a gynecomastia, small or large, leaves a large space that cannot be approximated without creating a marked deformity. The resulting dead space should therefore be drained rather than closed. Drains that are attached to negative-suction devices should be avoided. With the constant negative pressure, the skin adheres to the chest wall, resulting in a concave areola. The use of a Penrose drain is preferable. After the drain is removed, the dead space will fill with fibrous tissue.

The subcutaneous tissue is approximated using 2/0 plain catgut. The skin is approximated using continuous 4/0 monofilament absorbable sutures.

The gauze of the pressure dressing should have a cutout at its center to prevent flattening of the nipple [see Figure 11.44(B)].

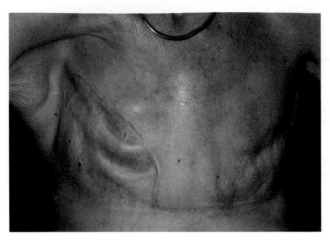

FIGURE 12.1

closed using a skin graft. The left-breast cancer was diagnosed in the late 1970s. It was treated by modified radical mastectomy. Both cancers were small. No axillary node involvement was detected in either axilla. The patient survived the breast cancers and died of heart failure. Today, her surgical treatment would be yet more conservative.

Figure 12.2

The patient in Figure 12.2 was treated for breast cancer in the early 1970s at the age of 55. The lesion measured 2 cm and was located in the medial quadrant at the 9 o'clock position. This patient was treated by extended radical mastectomy – that is, mastectomy, the resection of both pectoralis muscles and dissection of the axillary and internal mammary lymph nodes. The parasternal chest defect was

closed with fascia lata. The internal mammary and axillary lymph nodes were both free of disease. The photograph was taken with the patient at inspiration to emphasize the chest deformity created by this type of surgery.

Today, the patient would receive breast-conserving treatment: lumpectomy and axillary node dissection. Adjuvant chemotherapy and radiation therapy would be determined by pathology risk parameters – that is, intratumoral venous or arterial tumoral invasion, DNA index, HER-2/*neu* and p53 status.

Figure 12.3

The patient in Figure 12.3 was treated for breast cancer in mid-1990 with breast-conserving surgery. The lesion was located in the upper outer quadrant of the left breast. The surgical treatment consisted of lumpectomy and axillary node dissection, followed by radiation therapy. The arrows point to the scars. At 10 years from time of diagnosis, the patient was showing no evidence of disease.

Figure 12.4

The 61-year-old patient in Figure 12.4 was treated with a lumpectomy and level I axillary dissection for a 1-cm infiltrating ductal carcinoma tumor located in the retroareolar area. Because the tumor was attached to the nipple (causing nipple retraction), the nipple and areola were excised in block with the lesion. The arrow points to the scar from the axillary node dissection. This patient received adjuvant radiation therapy and tamoxifen.

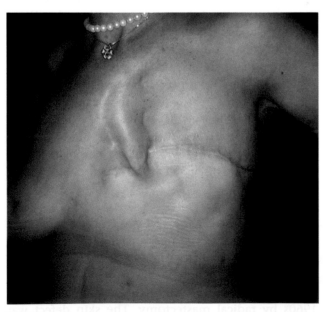

FIGURE 12.2

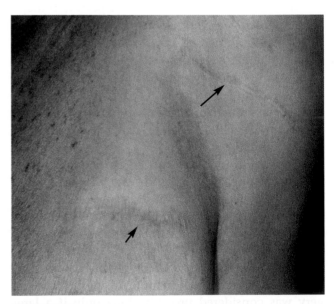

FIGURE 12.3

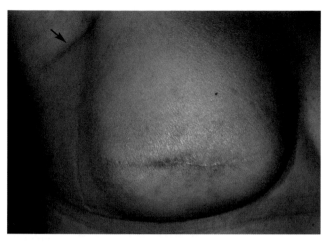

FIGURE 12.4

APPLIED SURGICAL ANATOMY OF THE BREAST

Topographically, the surgical anatomy of the breast corresponds to the anatomy of the chest wall and axilla.

Overall Structure

In an adult female, the breast occupies the interval between the second or third rib (superior boundary) and the six or seventh rib (inferior boundary). The lateral border of the sternum marks the medial boundary of the breast. Laterally, the breast extends to the mid axillary line, from which point it continues upward into the axilla as an extension – the so-called tail of Spence.

The posterior boundary of the breast is the posterior layer of the superficial pectoral fascia and the pectoralis major muscle. Between the posterior layer of this fascia and the posterior surface of the breast is a thin layer of adipose tissue.

At the anterior surface of the breast, centered, the nipple is surrounded by pigmented skin called the areola. In nulliparous patients, the nipple is located at the level of the fourth rib (or lower in patients with pendulous breasts).

The glandular portion of the breast is covered on its anterior and posterior surfaces by adipose tissue. The subcutaneous tissue takes the form of lobules held within the extensions of the suspensory ligaments of the breast (Cooper's ligaments).

The skin of the breast receives its sensory nerve supply from the fourth through the sixth intercostal nerves.

Muscles

The most important muscles in the region of the breast (as related to a modified radical mastectomy) are the pectoralis major and minor, the latissimus dorsi, the serratus anterior, and the subscapular.

PECTORALIS MAJOR MUSCLE

Figure 12.5

The pectoralis major originates in the sternal half of the clavicle, the sternal surface and the anterior surface of the first through the sixth rib, and the fascia of the external oblique muscle. It inserts into the lateral lip of the bicipital groove of the humerus as a small tendon resulting from the convergence of the fibers originating from the clavicle, the sternum, and the external oblique fascia.

The pectoralis major obtains its blood supply from the thoracoacromial artery, a branch of the thoracic artery. It is innervated by branches of the medial pectoral nerve for the clavicular portion and from the lateral pectoral nerve for the sternal and the external oblique portion (see Figure 12.11 later in this chapter).

The pectoralis major adducts the arm.

PECTORALIS MINOR MUSCLE

Figure 12.6

The pectoralis minor is located beneath the pectoralis major muscle. Its origin is digitations arising from the anterior surface of the third, fourth, and fifth ribs. From those three origins, the muscle fibers converge to insert at the medial and superior surface of the coracoid process of the scapula.

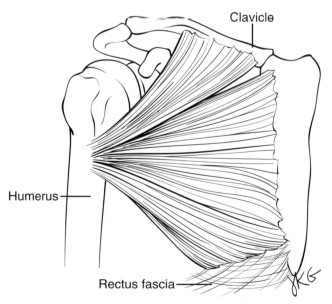

FIGURE 12.5

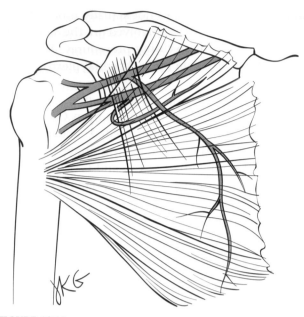

FIGURE 12.11

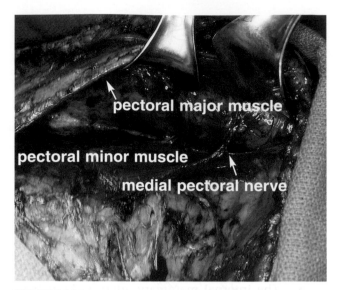

FIGURE 12.12

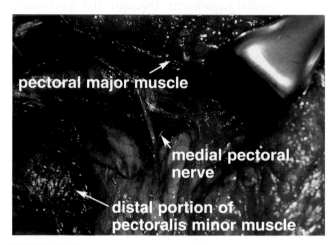

FIGURE 12.13

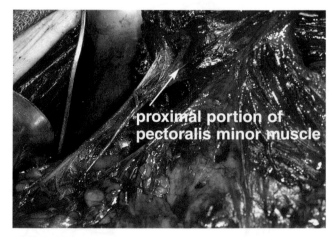

FIGURE 12.14

On its descent to the chest, the lateral pectoral nerve courses between the pectoralis major and minor muscles, runs along the medial border of the pectoralis minor, and provides branches to the sternal and costoabdominal insertions of the pectoralis major muscle. Injury to those branches results in atrophy of lower and inner portions of the pectoralis major. (Although the nerve runs along the medial border of the pectoralis minor, it is called the "lateral pectoral nerve" because its origin is in the lateral cord of the brachial plexus.)

Figures 12.12 and 12.13

Figure 12.12 shows the relationship between the medial pectoral nerve and the pectoralis minor muscle. The nerve runs along the lateral border of the muscle and then loops upward and medially to innervate the clavicular insertion of the pectoralis major muscle. Injury to this nerve causes that portion of the pectoralis major to atrophy. To avoid that complication during a modified radical mastectomy, the pectoralis minor should be transected distal the nerve (Figure 12.13).

Figure 12.14

The transected pectoralis minor muscle is shown being retracted up to reveal its posterior surface and to demonstrate some branches of the medial pectoral nerve in that surface.

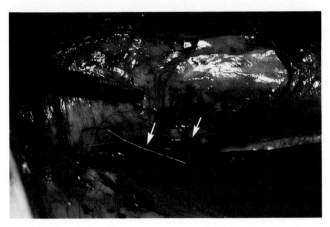

FIGURE 12.15

Figure 12.15
Occasionally, branches of the medial pectoral nerve pass through the pectoralis minor (arrows) to innervate muscle fascicles in the pectoralis major.

THORACODORSAL NERVE

The thoracodorsal nerve originates from the posterior cord of the brachial plexus. The nerve emerges in the axilla beneath the axillary vein medial to the subscapularis vessels (see Figure 12.100 later in this chapter). On its downward trajectory, it crosses through the lymph node–bearing tissues of the axilla, crosses over the subscapularis vessels, and (at that point) runs lateral to those vessels before entering the medial surface of the latissimus dorsi muscle.

Injury to the thoracodorsal nerve results in restriction of the internal rotation of the arm, not a major disability. If large suspicious nodes are present in the axilla, the nerve should be severed so that a more thorough nodal dissection can be performed.

LONG THORACIC NERVE

The long thoracic nerve originates from the fifth, sixth, and seventh spinal roots of the anterior cord of the brachial plexus (Figure 12.10). Its downward course crosses behind the axillary vein. The nerve emerges in the axilla, where it lies on the fascia of the serratus anterior muscle, staying close to the thoracic wall. (See Figures 12.93 and 12.100, later in this chapter.)

Injury to this nerve results in atrophy of the serratus anterior, which causes the scapula to rotate laterally and outward – the so-called winged scapula. To avoid injury to some branches of this nerve, the safest place to identify it is at the level of the second and third ribs (before it starts to give branches to the muscle fascicles of the serratus anterior).

Lymphatics and Lymph Nodes

The lymphatic vessels of the breast follow the blood vessels and drain to the lymph nodes of the axilla or to the internal mammary lymph nodes (or both).

Figure 12.16
The axillary nodes are divided into six groups. The groups are named to reflect the anatomic structures to which they are adjacent:

- The external mammary group lies over the axillary tail of the breast.
- The scapular group lies along the subscapular vessels.
- The axillary vein group lies along the axillary vein.
- The central axillary group lies beneath the lateral border of the pectoralis major muscle and below the lateral border of the pectoralis minor muscle.
- The subclavicular group (infraclavicular) lie at the costoclavicular junction (apical nodes).

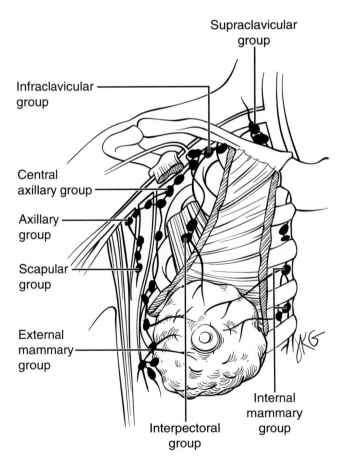

FIGURE 12.16

- The interpectoral (Rotter's) nodes lie between the pectoralis major and minor muscles along the lateral pectoral nerve.

Figure 12.17

The axillary lymph nodes are located within the axillary fat. From a surgical viewpoint, they are grouped into three levels:

- Level I nodes are located between the lateral border of the pectoralis minor muscle and the medial side of the latissimus dorsi muscle.
- Level II nodes are located behind the pectoralis minor muscle and below the axillary vein.
- Level III nodes, the highest group, are located medial to the medial border of the pectoralis minor muscle, along the medial and inferior surface of the axillary vein.

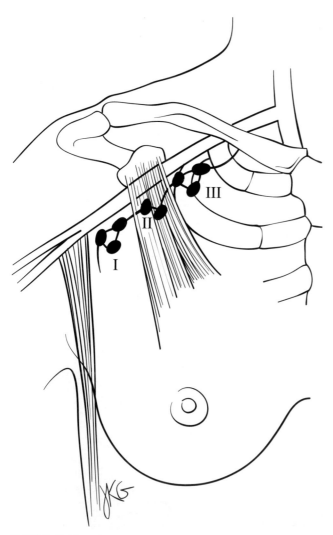

FIGURE 12.17

BREAST-CONSERVING SURGERY

The increased awareness of breast cancer among women and the technical advancements made in diagnosis and localization of breast lesions have resulted in a great number of breast cancers being diagnosed and operated on at an earlier stage. Surgical treatment for breast cancer has therefore moved from highly radical procedures to more conservative ones. With appropriate selection of patients, the survival rate with conservative procedures is reported to be comparable to that achieved with more radical surgery.

Breast-conserving surgeries include lumpectomy, excision of the axillary sentinel node, and axillary lymph node dissection with or without adjuvant radiotherapy. Only the surgical aspects of such treatments are discussed here. For the role of adjuvant radiotherapy in breast-conserving treatments, readers should consult the relevant textbooks.

Surgical Technique – Lumpectomy

"Lumpectomy" refers to the removal of a lump, benign or malignant. Although the connotation is somewhat different, the term is also used when the surgical procedure removes one or more clusters of malignant calcifications. When the lesion being removed is malignant, "lumpectomy" implies the removal of both the tumor and the surrounding tumor-free breast tissue.

Indications for a lumpectomy as breast-conserving treatment are

- a mammography finding of a small malignant lesion,
- planned excision of a cluster of microcalcifications, and
- treatment of T1 and T2 tumors. (For tumors larger than 3 cm, the author favors more radical surgery.)

Breast-conserving surgery is contraindicated for patients with small breasts, in whom wide, free margins cannot be obtained without causing breast deformity.

PREPARATION AND ANESTHESIA

A lumpectomy is usually done in an ambulatory setting under local infiltrative anesthesia and monitored intravenous sedation.

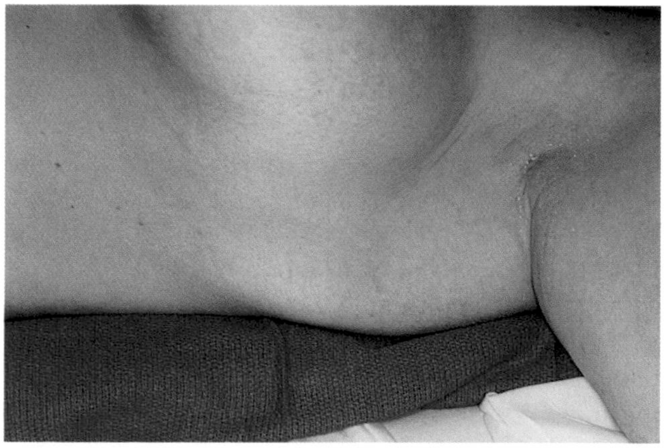

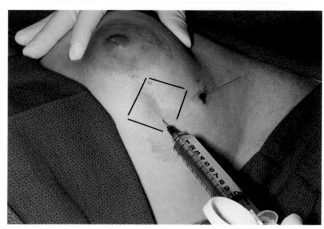

FIGURE 12.18

Figure 12.18

The patient is positioned eccentrically on the operating table, with the side being operated on near the edge of the table. If a patient has pendulous breasts, a pad placed under the ipsilateral side of the chest helps to elevate the latissimus dorsi muscle.

Figure 12.19

The local anesthetic agent of choice is bupivacaine. Bupivacaine is a long-acting local anesthetic. It takes its effect within two to five minutes after injection and lasts for four to five hours. The monitored sedation combines propofol, midazolam hydrochloride, and fentanyl citrate. Propofol is a hypnotic, which starts unconsciousness; midazolam causes amnesia; and fentanyl is a short-acting narcotic.

Injection of the local anesthetic agent occurs at two levels: in the subcutaneous tissue layer adjacent to the lesion and beyond the boundaries of the tumor or calcifications. The site of the planned incision is also injected. Although vasoconstrictors min-

imize intraoperative bleeding, they may give a false impression of complete hemostasis. They should not be added to the anesthetic agent.

Figure 12.20

When the lesion is located deep in the breast, additional local anesthetic should be injected into the breast parenchyma posterior to the lesion. The needle enters just above the breast crease (arrow) and is passed beyond the lesion parallel to the chest wall. The anesthetic agent is injected as the needle is being withdrawn. (Also see chapter 11, "Surgical Treatment of Benign Breast Lesions," Figure 11.52.)

INCISION

The skin incision should be planned so that it can be included in a re-excision should the patient require more radical surgery.

Figure 12.21

If the lesion is near the nipple–areola complex, a circumareolar incision is ideal. For lesions away from that area, the author favors radial incisions in the direction of the Kraissl's skin lines. Kraissl's lines are the dynamic skin lines of the breast that run perpendicular to the fibers of the underlying muscle. (Also see "Excision of a Single Benign Tumor" in chapter 11, "Surgical Treatment of Benign Breast Lesions.")

The incision is deepened through the subcutaneous tissue until breast tissue is encountered. Two skin flaps (an upper and a lower) are dissected in a tissue plane between the breast and the subcutaneous tissue. Dissection of the flaps should extend proximal and caudal to the estimated area of resection (arrows).

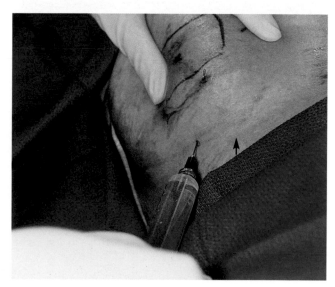

FIGURE 12.19

FIGURE 12.20

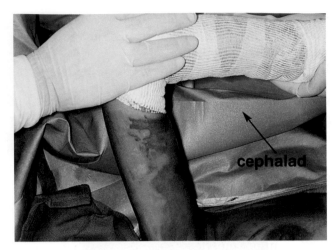

FIGURE 12.31

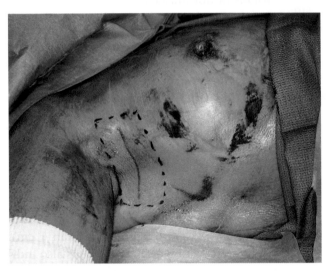

FIGURE 12.32

LEVEL I AND II AXILLARY DISSECTION – INCISION AND LEVEL I DISSECTION

A vertical incision should be avoided because it will inevitably heal with a hypertrophic scar or a keloid. The skin incision is made transversely, extending from the lateral border of the pectoralis muscle to the anterior border of the latissimus dorsi muscle (see Figure 12.32). The incision is made in the skin lines below the hairline to avoid maceration of the wound by perspiration.

Figure 12.33

The incision deepened through the skin, subcutaneous tissue, and axillary fascia.

Figure 12.33 shows the upper skin flap being developed. To facilitate dissection, the upper skin flap should be retracted cephalad and up. Dissection occurs in the plane between the subcutaneous tissue

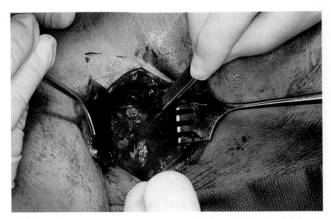

FIGURE 12.33

and the axillary fascia. To avoid an undesirable cosmetic result, as much of the subcutaneous tissue as possible should be preserved.

The lower flap is usually thicker than the upper one. It is fashioned by tapering it gradually down toward the chest wall.

Figure 12.34

Good exposure is essential. The anatomic landmarks in the dissection of the axilla include (anteriorly) the lateral border of the pectoralis major and minor muscle; (posteriorly) the latissimus dorsi muscle; (medially) the serratus anterior muscle; and (superiorly) the axillary vein, the intercostobrachial nerve, the thoracodorsal nerve, and the long thoracic nerve.

Once the skin flaps are complete, the superficial pectoral fascia is dissected to expose the pectoralis major muscle (arrow). The skeletonization of that muscle should extend far enough to accommodate a medium-sized retractor.

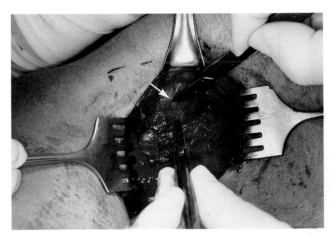

FIGURE 12.34

In Figure 12.34, the pectoralis major muscle is being retracted superiorly to expose the lateral border of the pectoralis minor muscle. When level I and level II axillary lymph nodes are all being excised, the pectoralis minor muscle should also be skeletonized. The dissection along that muscle is carried cephalad along the edge until the medial pectoral nerve is encountered.

The medial pectoral nerve arises from the medial trunk of the brachial plexus. It enters the axilla under the axillary vein and runs along the lateral edge of the pectoralis minor muscle. It then curves anteriorly along the belly of the muscle to give branches to the clavicular origin of the muscle. (See Figure 12.88 later in this section.) Injury to this nerve causes atrophy in the clavicular portion of the pectoralis major muscle.

Figure 12.35

The fascia of the latissimus dorsi (arrow) is incised along its lateral border to avoid injury to the thoracodorsal nerve. That nerve enters the muscle along its medial surface. When level II axillary nodes are being excised, dissection of the latissimus dorsi muscle should extend to its tendinous portion. The axillary vein is superior to the tendon, which functions as a landmark to identify the vein.

Figure 12.36

When the skeletonization of the pectoralis major and the latissimus dorsi muscles is complete, the axillary fat pad that bears the lymph nodes is exposed (A). The author prefers to start the axillary dissection caudal of this anatomic landmark that separates level I from level II nodes. The starting point of the dissection is arbitrary, but in general it should be done at the level of the fourth and fifth rib.

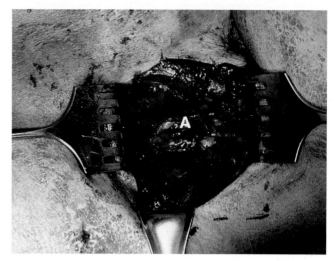

FIGURE 12.36

Figure 12.37

When traction is exerted on the lower skin flap, the surgeon can identify the most caudal portion of the axillary fat pad. Dissection commences at that point, cutting down through the clavipectoral fascia toward the serratus anterior muscle. Once the inferior-most site of the dissection has been established and incised, the dissection continues cephalad on that plane.

Better exposure of the axilla is obtained when the pectoralis major, pectoralis minor, and latissimus dorsi muscles are relaxed. Flexing the patient's arm at the elbow and internally rotating the still-abducted arm at the shoulder accomplishes the necessary relaxation (see Figure 12.31). To perform that maneuver, the second assistant holds the patient's arm at the elbow and hand. As the assistant flexes the patient's forearm and brings it forward, he or she pushes the elbow back in the direction of the patient's head.

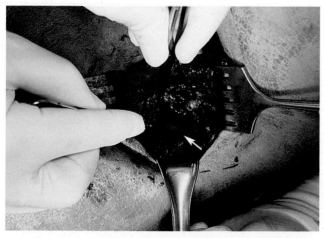

FIGURE 12.35

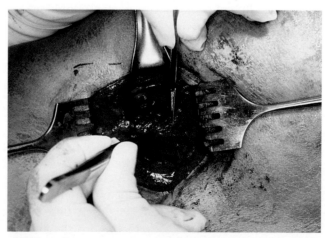

FIGURE 12.37

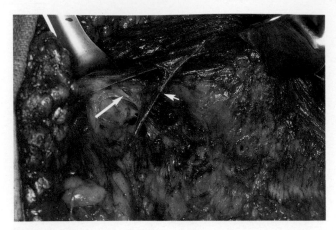

FIGURE 12.38

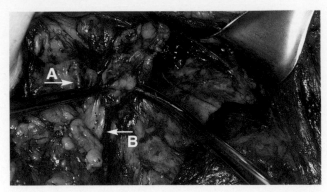

FIGURE 12.39

Figure 12.38

The dissection continues to the level at which the intercostobrachial nerve is encountered (small arrow). That nerve is the anatomic landmark that separates level I from level II.

The intercostobrachial nerve is a sensory nerve. It emerges to the axilla through the intercostal muscle and crosses the axilla (medial to lateral) giving a few sensory branches to the medial and posterior superior surfaces of the arm, the axilla, and the part of the back adjacent to the axilla. Unless suspicious metastatic nodes are present, an effort should be made to preserve the nerve. If it is cut, the patient will experience numbness along the medial aspect of the ipsilateral arm.

The intercostobrachial nerve is also an anatomic landmark that helps to identify the long thoracic nerve. That nerve (large arrow) runs along the chest wall.

LEVEL I AND II AXILLARY DISSECTION – LEVEL I EXCISION

If the clinical indication is to excise only level I lymph nodes, then dissection stops here, and the axillary fat pad is serially clamped and transected.

A suture is placed in the proximal margin to situate the specimen.

LEVEL I AND II AXILLARY DISSECTION – LEVEL II DISSECTION

To extend the dissection to level II, the axillary vein must first be identified. The axillary vein can be found approximately 1–2 cm superior to the intercostobrachial nerve, lying anterior and inferior to the artery. Finding the vein may be more difficult in obese patients. In such cases, feeling for the axillary artery's pulse will help to identify the location.

Starting the level II dissection along the axillary vein is the safer course. Dissection starts laterally near the tendon of the latissimus dorsi muscle and continues medially, holding back from the vein to avoid trauma.

Figure 12.39

The first afferent branch encountered is the subscapularis vein (arrow A). That vein is located in a deeper plane. It is a landmark to the thoracodorsal nerve, which is found medial to the vein (arrow B). On its downward course, the nerve crosses over the subscapular vein and then travels lateral to it before entering the latissimus dorsi muscle along its medial surface.

LEVEL I AND II AXILLARY DISSECTION – LEVEL II EXCISION

The level II axillary lymph nodes are located behind the pectoralis minor muscle. Dissection continues medially toward the lateral border of that muscle. Because the pectoralis minor muscle is spared in breast-conserving surgery, the muscle is retracted medially and upward for excision of the level II nodes.

With the thoracodorsal and the long thoracic nerves both in view, the fat-bearing lymph nodes are dissected off the vein. Slightly open dissecting scissors push the fat downward until the specimen is removed (see Figure 12.96).

To situate the specimen, a silk suture is placed in its apex, marking its most proximal portion.

INDICATIONS FOR LEVEL III LYMPH NODE DISSECTION

The axillary lymph nodes at level III are the subclavicular nodes – also called the apical nodes of the axilla. Dissection of the level III axillary lymph nodes is seldom indicated in breast-conserving surgery. More commonly, such a dissection forms part of a

modified radical mastectomy. Dissection in the latter context is fully discussed in "Surgical Technique – Modified Radical Mastectomy" later in this chapter. Here, a level III dissection is discussed in the context of breast-conserving surgery.

Indications for dissection of the level III axillary nodes are

- a finding of involved or suspicious lymph nodes during dissection at levels I and II, and
- a large cancer in a patient who refuses mastectomy.

LEVEL III AXILLARY DISSECTION

Figure 12.40

The anatomic landmarks for level III are (superior) the axillary vein (A), (inferior) the medial border of the pectoralis minor (B), and (medial) the ligament of Halsted (arrow). (Figure 12.40 shows the left axilla.)

To facilitate the level III dissection, the patient's arm, still abducted, is extended upward and cephalad as the elbow is brought caudal (forearm flexed). This maneuver relaxes the pectoralis major muscle and provides better access to level III (see Figure 12.31).

The pectoralis minor muscle is skeletonized with great care to avoid injury to the lateral and medial pectoral nerves. Using the index finger of the non-dominant hand, the surgeon dissects the muscle from its posterior surface and retracts it laterally and down. The clavipectoral fascia is incised, and the axillary vein is exposed.

With dissecting scissors kept slightly open, the dissection progresses by cutting and "pushing" the fat-bearing nodal tissue until the level III is completely removed.

AXILLARY DISSECTION, ALL LEVELS – CLOSURE

Before closure, the wound is irrigated with warm distilled water to remove loose particles of fat and tissue. The subcutaneous tissue is closed using interrupted sutures of 2/0 plain catgut. The skin is closed with a continuous suture of 4/0 absorbable monofilament.

A drain is inserted and attached to a negative-suction device. A pressure dressing is applied.

Figure 12.41

Figure 12.41 shows the postoperative appearance of the axilla following an axillary node dissection. The contour of the axilla is preserved. (The arrow points to the scar.)

COMPLICATIONS

The possible complications of an axillary lymph node dissection are

- injury to the axillary vein,
- arm edema, and
- injury to the thoracodorsal, long thoracic, and medial and lateral pectoral nerves.

Of all those complications, arm edema is the most likely, whether the procedure was part of a modified radical mastectomy or of breast-conserving surgery. The incidence of arm edema following an axillary node dissection can be minimized or prevented by meticulous dissection that avoids trauma to the axillary vein, and by teaching and encourag-

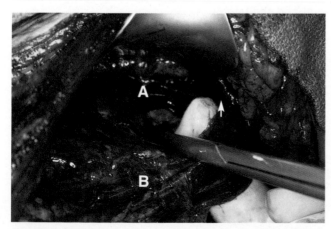

FIGURE 12.40

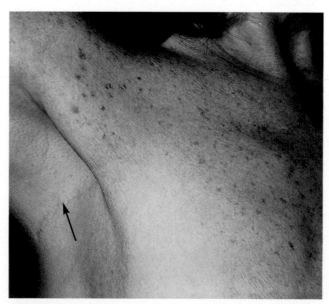

FIGURE 12.41

ing the patient to practice postoperative arm and shoulder exercises.

Nerve injuries resulting from an axillary dissection are discussed in "Surgical Technique – Modified Radical Mastectomy" later in this chapter.

Surgical Technique – Excision of the Sentinel Node

At the end of the nineteenth century, Halsted described the surgical technique for a radical mastectomy. Since then, a major shift to lesser procedures has occurred in breast cancer treatment. Management of the axilla has also changed from total axillary dissection, to excision of the level I and II lymph nodes, and (more recently) to excision of the sentinel node in the axilla.

The sentinel node is the axillary node at which lymph flow from the breast arrives first. In keeping with the theory that lymph flow is linear, tumor cells in the lymphatic channels are expected to reach the sentinel node before spreading to the other nodes. Because complete management of breast cancer depends on the status of the axillary nodes, excision of the sentinel node for biopsy has become increasingly accepted as a means to stage the disease.

Excision of the sentinel node is a multidisciplinary procedure. It requires the combined efforts of nuclear medicine (to inject a radioactive mapping agent), the surgeon (to inject a mapping dye and to localize and excise the node), and the pathologist to determine on frozen section whether metastasis is present.

INDICATIONS FOR SENTINEL NODE DISSECTION

Indications for a sentinel node dissection are

- certain cases of DCIS, such as the high-grade and comedo necrosis types;
- cases of large tumors (such as T1 and T2) with no clinically palpable nodes;
- cases of minimally invasive carcinomas (micrometastasis); and
- cases of histologically favorable invasive carcinomas with a low probability of metastasis (for example, tubular, medullary, colloid).

Regardless of the size of the cancer, excision of the sentinel node for staging is contraindicated in patients with palpable suspicious nodes.

APPLIED ANATOMY OF THE BREAST LYMPHATICS

In general, the role of the lymphatic system is to clear cellular debris. In the breast, that role is the same: to drain the debris of an inflammatory process or to transport emboli of cancer cells to the axillary basin. In either of those processes, the axillary lymph nodes become enlarged owing to reactive or metastatic lymphoadenopathy.

Lymph flow from the breast acini to the axillary lymph nodes is not direct from lesion to lymph nodes. Rather, the flow travels from the acini to connecting channels that drain to a subareolar lymphatic plexus and thence to the sentinel node. Basic knowledge of the embryology provides a better understanding.

The breast is an organ of the ectoderm that appears early in the development of the embryo. By the sixth week, a thickening of the ectoderm appears on each side of the chest and the abdomen, extending from the axilla to the pubis and forming a ridge (the "milk line" – see chapter 6, "Role of the Clinician – Female Breast," Figure 6.24). In human embryos of about 10 mm, the ridge remains a localized thickening in the region of the future breast.

Figure 12.42
In the late stages of gestation, the breast has already formed its lactiferous ducts and secretory lobules. When the initial breast bud invaginates, the lymphatics of the skin are carried deep into the breast parenchyma ending in the acini and periacinar area of the lobule.

Because carcinoma of the breast originates in the perilobular segment of the acini, and the lymphatic vessels are the path of metastasis, metastasis progresses in a centrifugal fashion from the periacinar and duct regions into larger lymphatic vessels that then flow into two main lymphatic trunks, the medial and the lateral (A).

In their courses to the areolar region, the two trunks receive secondary tributary vessels. The lateral trunk receives the lymphatic tributaries that drain the superior quadrants of the breast. The medial trunk receives the tributaries that drain the inferior quadrants. The two lymphatic trunks converge in the retroareolar area to form a circumareolar plexus, the subareolar lymphatic plexus of Sappey (B).

By Sappey's original description (later confirmed by Rouvière, also a French anatomist), the circumareolar plexus constitutes a lymphatic way station before draining to the axillary sentinel node (C). Rouvière's contribution was to describe not only the

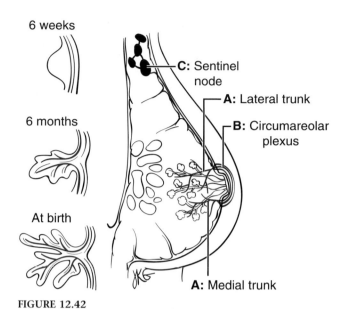

FIGURE 12.42

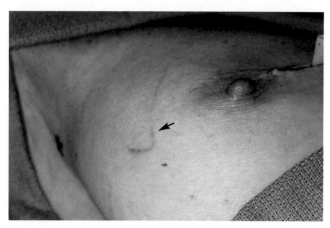

FIGURE 12.43

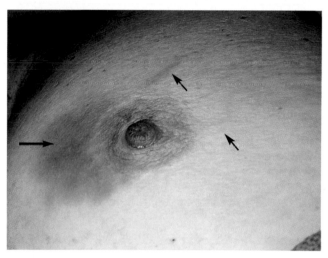

FIGURE 12.44

lymphatic path to the axilla but also that to the internal mammary lymph nodes.

Testut and Jacob (other French anatomists) described two lymphatic chains, one superficial and one deep. The superficial chain runs in the subcutaneous tissue. Some parts drain into the axillary nodes and some into the supraclavicular and internal mammary nodes. The deep chain ("intercostal chain," from its location between the intercostal muscles) has two trunks. One drains posteriorly to the pleura, and the other, anteriorly to the internal mammary chain. The posterior trunk of the deep chain may explain metastatic breast disease in the pleura and lung.

Although most of the lymph-collecting vessels terminate in the axillary nodes (Figure 12.43), some afferent lymph vessels drain into the nodes of the internal mammary chain (Figure 12.44 [arrows]). Approximately 95% of the vessels are estimated to drain to the axilla; only a small fraction, about 5%, drain to the internal mammary chain.

Locally recurrent carcinoma of the breast usually occurs along the mastectomy scar. Locally recurrent breast carcinoma may therefore be conceived as being attributable to the presence of dormant malignant cells within the dermal lymphatics in the periareolar network. That may be why an ample excision of skin in the periareolar region during a mastectomy helps to minimize local recurrence.

Figures 12.43 and 12.44

In Figure 12.43 (right breast), the site of greater lymphatic uptake is marked in the skin of the axilla. Dye was injected into the subcutaneous tissue medial border of the areola. The subareolar plexus is stained by dye and a lymphatic vessel leading toward the sentinel node is similarly stained (arrow).

In Figure 12.44 (right breast), the dye was injected on the lateral border of the areola. The subareolar plexus (of Sappey [large arrow]) and lymphatic vessels leading toward the internal mammary nodes are stained (small arrows).

MAPPING THE SENTINEL NODE

The sentinel node can be mapped in any of three ways:

- Intraparenchymal injection of technetium-labeled sulfur colloid
- Intraparenchymal injection of isosulfan blue dye
- Intraparenchymal injection of a combination of both agents

The use of the dual agents is preferable because accuracy in detecting the sentinel node is optimized.

The optimal time for injection of the technetium colloid solution depends on the solution's particle size. The larger the particles, the longer they take to reach the sentinel node. Small particles (filtered) in the range of 10–200 μ take, on average, three to four hours to reach the sentinel node. Isosulfan blue dye is injected in the operating room just before the induction of anesthesia.

One contentious issue in sentinel node mapping is the site for the injection of the mapping agents. Intraparenchymal injection of the dye not only retards transit of the dye, it also obscures the operative field. Drainage may take even longer in patients whose normal lymphatic drainage has been disrupted by prior surgical biopsies, extensive injury, burns, or previous reconstructive surgery to the breast.

The author prefers to inject the mapping agents into the subcutaneous tissue just below the dermis, close to the areola margin (*Sappey's plexus*). When isosulfan blue dye is injected into that area, it takes approximately fifteen to thirty minutes to reach the sentinel node.

Figures 12.45 and 12.46

The patient in Figures 12.45 and 12.46 had undergone two surgical procedures on the same day. Both procedures were for clusters of malignant microcalcifications. A lesion at 10 o'clock (upper scar) was cribriform DCIS with tumor-free margins. A lesion at 9 o'clock (lower scar) was a comedo DCIS with tumor close to one of the margins. For that reason, a re-excision of breast tissue and excision of the sentinel node were recommended.

Mapping dye was injected into the medial side of the areola away from the site of the lesion. Figure 12.45 shows the progress of the dye from the site of the injection through the lateral quadrants of the breast toward the axilla (arrow) in the direction of the sentinel node (marked with an *X*). The time from injection of the dye to visualization in the skin was fifteen minutes.

The scar was re-excised (Figure 12.46), and the incision deepened through the subcutaneous tissue layer down to the breast-tissue plane. The dye is already seen in the subcutaneous tissue on the side opposite to the injection.

The dye does not stain the breast parenchyma. Also, regardless of the site of injection – medial or lateral to the areola margin – the dye always pro-

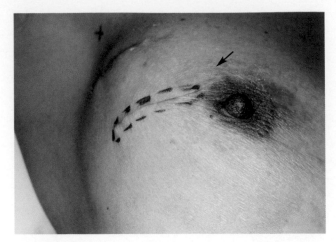

FIGURE 12.45

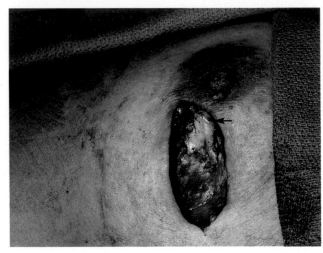

FIGURE 12.46

gresses to the sentinel node. The next few figures illustrate it.

Figure 12.47

The lesion was located in the lower inner quadrant of the left breast (small arrow). Dye was injected in the lateral margin of the areola (large arrow).

Figures 12.48 and 12.49

The dye can be seen to be progressing through the lymphatic vessel running on the subcutaneous tissue of the superior skin flap (arrows).

Figure 12.50

The dye has reached the sentinel node (arrow). Confirmation of the sentinel node was provided by both the blue staining and an increased uptake of the radioactive agent in vivo.

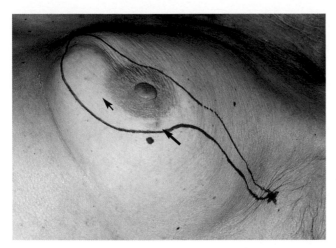

FIGURE 12.47

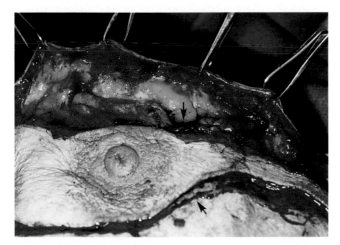

FIGURE 12.48

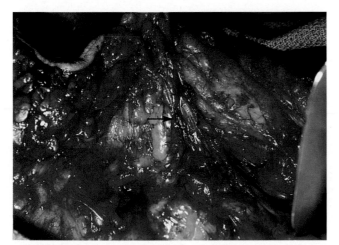

FIGURE 12.49

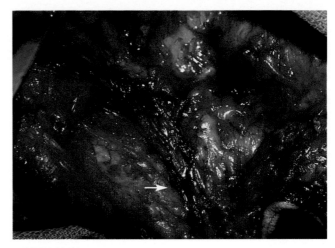

FIGURE 12.50

PREPARATION

Unlike axillary node dissection, sentinel node excision can proceed in an ambulatory surgical facility under local anesthesia and monitored sedation. However, infiltration of the local anesthetic agent distorts the operative field. For that reason, general anesthesia may be preferable.

Figure 12.51 and 12.52

The patient's ipsilateral arm is abducted and placed on an arm board at right angles to the body. A small pillow placed beneath the patient's back elevates the latissimus dorsi muscle.

The area registering the highest radioactivity count is marked on the skin of the axilla.

If lumpectomy and excision of the sentinel node are done during the same surgical intervention, the lumpectomy is done first. This approach reduces the possibility of malignant cells contaminating the axilla. It also reduces the "shine through" effect from high uptake of radiocolloid in the area of the lesion.

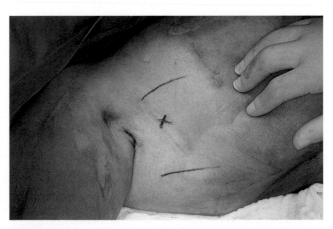

FIGURE 12.51

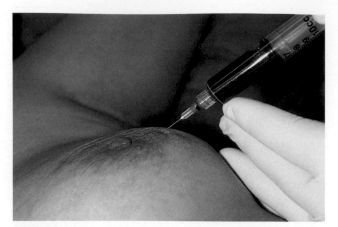

FIGURE 12.52

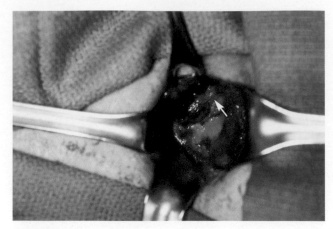

FIGURE 12.54

Isosulfan blue dye is injected into the subdermis of the periareolar area before the induction of anesthesia. A waiting period (fifteen to twenty minutes) should elapse between the time of the injection and the start of the procedure.

The skin of the anterolateral chest wall, the breast, the upper arm, and the axilla is prepared with an antiseptic solution.

The lateral border of the pectoralis major and latissimus dorsi muscles are marked as guidelines. To avoid a hypertrophic scar caused by skin perspiration, the incision is made below the level of sudoriparous glands.

The incision for a sentinel node biopsy should be smaller than that for a formal axillary node dissection. If the pathology report indicates the need for a complete axillary dissection, the excision can be extended at that time.

Figures 12.53 and 12.54

The skin incision is continued through the subcutaneous tissue. At that level, the skin flaps are com-

pleted by sharp dissection and are separated using rake retractors. The incision is deepened through the clavipectoral fascia (Figure 12.53, arrow) to enter to the axillary space. Often, the stained lymph node and an afferent stained lymphatic vessel can be seen upon entering the axilla (Figure 12.54).

Figures 12.55 and 12.56

Figure 12.55 shows the stained afferent lymph vessel draining in the direction of a partially blue-stained lymph node. Regardless of whether the node is stained, confirmation that it is the sentinel node should be checked by its radiocolloid uptake (which should be increased). A node with an in vivo radioactivity count at least 5×–10× higher than the background level marks the sentinel node even when it is unstained (Figure 12.56).

Figure 12.57

The gross specimen in Figure 12.57 was confirmed as the sentinel node because of the increased

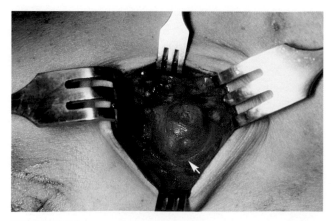

FIGURE 12.53

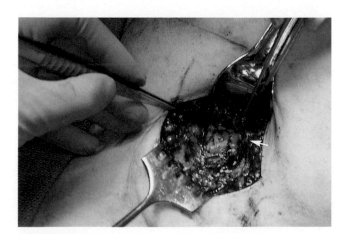

FIGURE 12.55

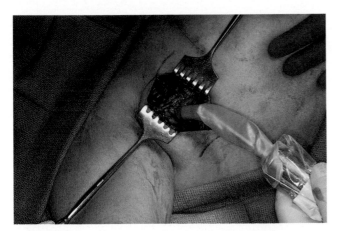

FIGURE 12.56

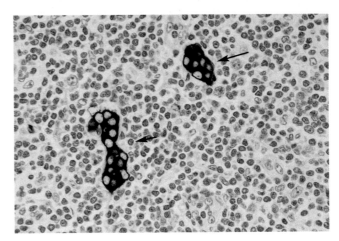

FIGURE 12.58

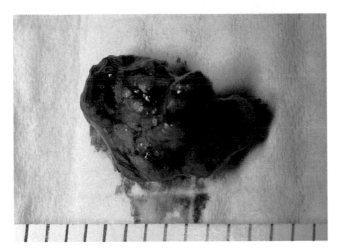

FIGURE 12.57

radioactivity measured in vivo and ex vivo. The specimen should be sent for frozen-section examination.

The operative field is again probed and any other nodes showing increased radioactivity should also be removed. Those nodes are sent for permanent sections.

Figure 12.58

The pathologist's role in breast cancer management by sentinel node biopsy comes into play when the specimen is analyzed on frozen sections. The specimen is processed by serial sectioning using both hematoxylin–eosin and immunohistochemical (IHC) cytokeratin staining. The IHC technique uses antibodies to cytokeratins to identify epithelial cells in the specimen. Those cells are presumed to represent metastasis from the breast (arrows). If the sentinel node is negative on frozen and on permanent sections, no further axillary nodes dissection is indicated.

When a diagnosis of metastasis is made from the frozen sections, a more extensive axillary node dis-

section is performed immediately. If the frozen sections are negative for metastasis, but pathology is then diagnosed on the permanent sections, a more extensive axillary dissection is indicated. The patient will have to return for more surgery.

CLOSURE

Hemostasis is completed, and the axillary cavity is irrigated with warm water to remove small clots that may hide bleeding.

Figure 12.59

The subcutaneous tissue is closed with interrupted sutures of 2/0 catgut. The skin incision is closed with an absorbable monofilament suture. A Penrose drain is inserted into the axillary cavity. The drain is usually removed in 24–48 hours, depending the amount of drainage.

Before being discharged from the hospital, the patient should be advised that her urine will be stained

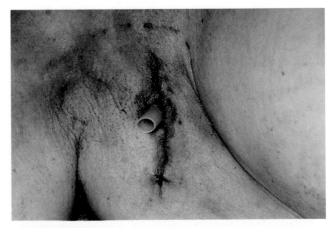

FIGURE 12.59

blue for the next 24 hours. The skin tattoo from the dye injection remains for two to three months.

COMPLICATIONS

Excision of the sentinel node causes practically no morbidity. Complications such as paresthesia in the skin of the axilla, wound infection, seroma, and acute or chronic lymphedema can occur, but they occur with lesser frequency than with a formal axillary dissection.

TOTAL MASTECTOMY

In a total mastectomy, only the breast and a few level I lymph nodes are excised. The lymph nodes are removed to insure complete removal of the tail of Spence, which extends into the axilla. The total mastectomy approach contrasts with that of the modified radical mastectomy, in which not only the breast, but most levels of the axillary lymph nodes *and* the pectoralis minor muscle are removed.

The surgical steps in a total mastectomy are

- elevation of two skin flaps.
- dissection of the breast from the pectoralis major muscle.
- skeletonization of the lateral border of the pectoralis major muscle.
- incision of the clavipectoral fascia to enter the axilla and remove the tail of Spence and a few level I lymph nodes.
- dissection of the breast from its chest wall attachment near the latissimus dorsi muscle.
- wound closure.

The indications for a total mastectomy are

- a combination of high risk for breast cancer plus extensive findings of pre-malignant mastopathy such as lobular carcinoma in situ (LCIS, "lobular neoplasia") in a patient who carries the BRCA1 and BRCA2 genes (Figure 12.60). In such cases, the procedure is prophylactic.
- multifocal, multicentric, ductal or lobular carcinoma in situ (Figure 12.61).
- locally recurrent carcinoma after breast-conserving surgery (Figure 12.62)
- extensive involvement of the breast. This palliative procedure is also called a "cleansing mastectomy" or "toilette mastectomy" (Figures 12.63, 12.64, and 12.65).

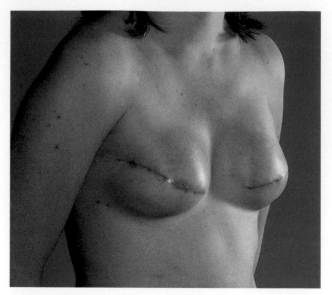

FIGURE 12.60

Figure 12.60

A set of high risk factors led the 37-year-old patient in Figure 12.60 to have a prophylactic bilateral mastectomy and an immediate breast reconstruction. Her mother had been diagnosed with breast carcinoma at age 34 and had died at age 36. Her sister had been diagnosed with breast cancer at age 36. The patient had experienced menarche at age 11 and became parous at later than the average age. During genetic counseling, she tested positive for the BRCA1 gene.

After further counseling and several surgical opinions, bilateral mastectomy with immediate reconstruction was performed. Pathology analysis of the specimens revealed ductal hyperplasia with atypia in the right breast and lobular carcinoma in situ in the left breast.

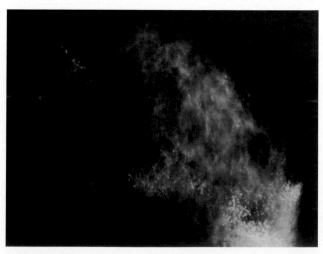

FIGURE 12.61

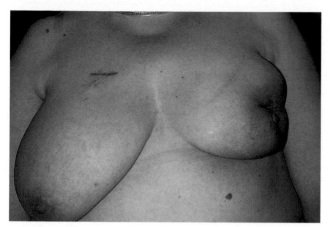

FIGURE 12.62

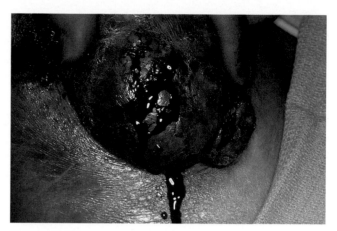

FIGURE 12.63

Figure 12.61

A mammogram in the cranial–caudal (CC) view images extensive, branching microcalcifications in all the quadrants of a patient's breast. A total mastectomy and excision of the sentinel node was done.

Figure 12.62

When a carcinoma recurs locally in patients treated with breast-conserving surgery, a total mastectomy is indicated. Because radiotherapy typically results in frail skin, the wound was closed with a latissimus dorsi skin flap (see chapter 13, "Role of the Plastic Surgeon").

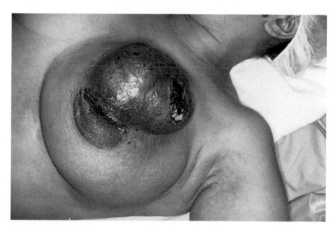

FIGURE 12.64

Figures 12.63, 12.64, and 12.65

The patient in Figure 12.63 had fungating breast carcinoma with extensive necrosis that was eroding the intratumoral blood vessels – a dramatic clinical presentation. To stop the bleeding, the wound was packed in the operating room. The patient was then treated with a few cycles of chemotherapy to downstage the disease in preparation for a "cleansing mastectomy."

The tumor decreased in size after four cycles of chemotherapy (Figure 12.64). The extent of the mass is clearly demonstrated in this photograph taken in the operating room at the time of the scheduled mastectomy (Figure 12.65).

The patient's skin defect was closed using a skin graft. The term "cleansing mastectomy" or "toilette mastectomy" is used when the procedure is palliative in nature. Fortunately, increasing patient awareness means that cases like this are nowadays seldom seen.

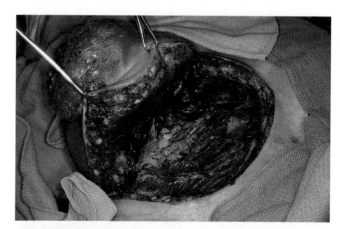

FIGURE 12.65

Surgical Technique – Total Mastectomy

PREPARATION

The patient is placed supine on the operating table, eccentrically positioned with the side to be op-

erated on near the edge of the table. The arm is abducted and placed on an arm board. Folded sheets are placed under the ipsilateral side of the chest, elevating its lateral aspect to better demarcate the latissimus dorsi muscle.

The skin of the anterior thorax, axilla, neck, arm, and upper abdomen is prepared with an antiseptic solution, and the area is draped.

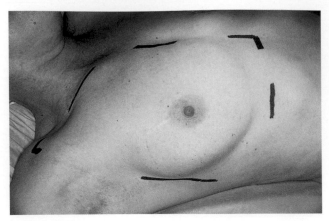

FIGURE 12.66

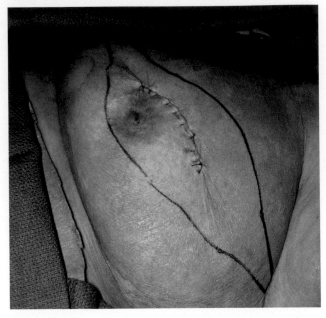

FIGURE 12.68

Figure 12.66

The extent of the skin-flap dissection is mapped. On the vertical axis, the dissection extends to the clavicle (superiorly) and to the low costal margin (inferiorly). On the horizontal axis, it extends from the lateral border of the sternum (medially) to the anterior border of the latissimus dorsi muscles (laterally).

Figure 12.67

The forearm is covered with stockinet to keep that part of the limb sterile in case the arm has to be moved during the axillary dissection. This technique becomes even more useful in a modified radical mastectomy, facilitating the axillary dissection should access to the apical nodes be required.

Figure 12.68

When possible, the skin incision should be fashioned transversely across the chest wall. A mastec-

tomy scar running in that direction is cosmetically more acceptable to the patient and allows her to wear V-neck clothing.

The incision extends from just lateral to the lateral border of the sternum to the anterior border of the latissimus dorsi muscle. The incision includes the nipple, the tumor site, and the biopsy incision if a biopsy has previously been done. A transverse incision is always technically feasible when the tumor is located on the 3 o'clock or 9 o'clock radius, or even at the 6 o'clock or 12 o'clock position, with the lesion close to the areola margin.

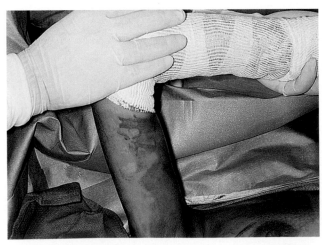

FIGURE 12.67

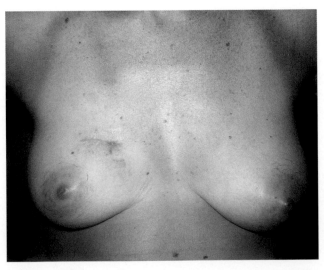

FIGURE 12.69A

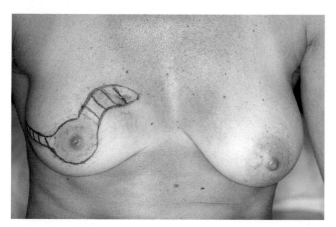

FIGURE 12.69B

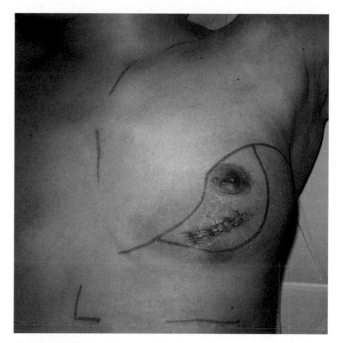

FIGURE 12.70

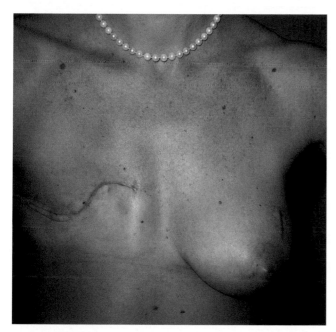

FIGURE 12.69C

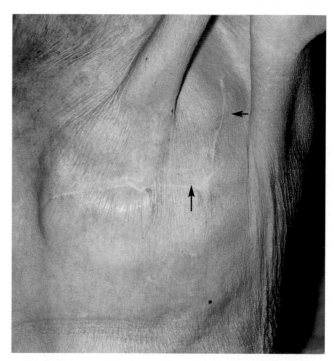

FIGURE 12.71

Figure 12.69A, B, C

A transverse incision is also feasible when the lesion is located in the upper or the lower quadrant of the breast. This patient's lesion was located in the upper inner quadrant of the left breast (A). The incision was fashioned in the form of an *S* (B). When the wound was closed, the scar lay transverse across the chest (C).

Figure 12.70

In Figure 12.70, the patient's lesion was located in the lower quadrant on the midline. An oblique scar resulted from the marked incision.

Figures 12.71 and 12.72

In patients with large, pendulous breasts, a transverse incision may result in a "doggy ear," if the closure is not appropriately designed. The patient is un-

comfortable because the excess skin rubs against the inner surface of the arm (Figure 12.72). To avoid the problem, the skin incision should be curved toward the axilla, below the axillary hairline. It should commence at about the fifth or six rib, near the lateral border of the sternum medially. It should end at the edge of the latissimus dorsi muscle at the level of the second or third rib.

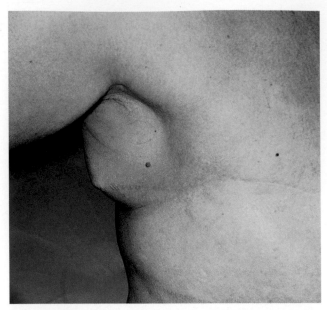

FIGURE 12.72

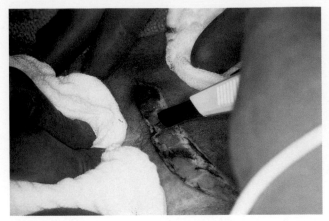

FIGURE 12.73

INCISION

The author favors the Shaw hemostatic scalpel over conventional steel blades. The hemostatic scalpel reduces operating time by minimizing blood loss and excessive tying or coagulation of small blood vessels. [See "Suggested Reading," Pilnik and Steichen (1986).]

The skin incision is fashioned in an ellipse that includes the nipple–areola complex and the scar from the biopsy. It extends from the edge of the latissimus dorsi muscle to about 1 cm from the lateral border of the sternum. Extension of the incision to the level of the sternum should be avoided. The skin on that part of the chest is not lax, and a keloid in that portion of the wound will be the result.

Figure 12.73

The skin flap should incorporate a thin layer of adjacent subcutaneous tissue.

Figure 12.74

The incision is deepened through the skin and dermis to just below the superficial layer of the superficial fascia. This fascia is very thin, but it is a definite anatomic structure. Because large axial vessels lie deep to the superficial fascia, dissecting deep to that plane may cause excessive bleeding.

Figure 12.75A and 12.75B

Superior and inferior skin flaps are elevated. The upper skin flap reaches to the level of the clavicle, and the lower flap is extended to the edge of the costal margin.

An even skin flap can be obtained if the scalpel blade is positioned parallel to the flap during the dissection (A). The proper positioning is accomplished by the surgeon applying downward traction on the breast with the non-dominant hand and the assistant applying traction to the flap at a 90-degree angle to the chest wall (B).

As the skin flaps are being dissected medially near the sternum, a few perforator veins will be encountered. These large vessels should be ligated rather than coagulated.

Figure 12.76

To facilitate dissection of the lower skin flap, the surgeon should change position, coming around the

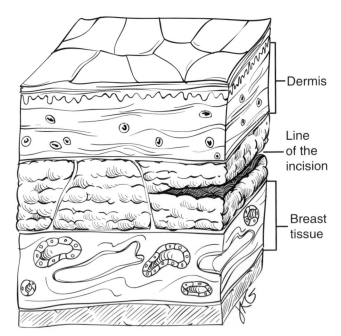

FIGURE 12.74

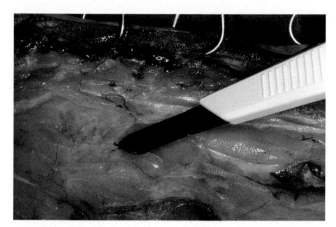

FIGURE 12.75A

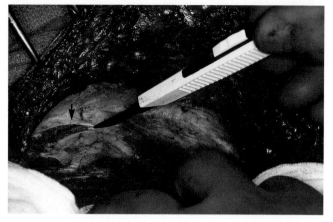

FIGURE 12.77

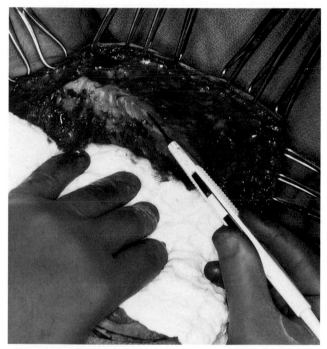

FIGURE 12.75B

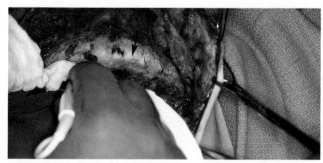

FIGURE 12.76

patient's abducted arm to face in the direction of the patient's feet.

The lower skin flap is developed in the same fashion as the upper one. The dissection extends down toward the costal margin to approximately 4–5 cm below the inframammary fold (arrow).

Figure 12.77

Lymphatic drainage of the lower inner quadrant of the breast is to the epigastric lymph nodes. Those lymph nodes drain to the upper abdomen and to the liver. When the lesion is an infiltrating carcinoma located in the lower inner quadrant of the breast, the rectus muscle fascia should be excised (arrow). Excision of the rectus fascia is not otherwise necessary during a total mastectomy.

Figure 12.78

When the lower and upper skin flaps are complete, dissection continues laterally toward the latissimus dorsi muscle (arrow). When the muscle is reached, dissection progresses cephalad along the lateral edge of the muscle and continues upward until the tendinous portion of the muscle is identified.

The tendon of the latissimus dorsi muscle constitutes the "floor" of the axilla. It is the anatomic landmark that helps to locate the axillary vein before axillary dissection begins.

EXCISION

Figure 12.79

Removal of the breast commences medially near the lateral border of the sternum in a plane deep to the superficial pectoral fascia. The line of the excision extends from the level of the second rib (superiorly) to the seventh rib (inferiorly) just medial to the lateral border of the sternum.

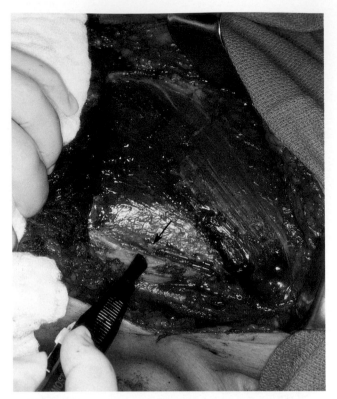

FIGURE 12.78

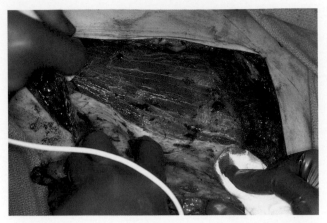

FIGURE 12.80

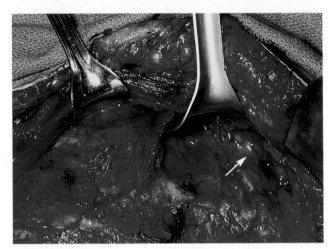

FIGURE 12.81

and the deep pectoral fascia and the clavipectoral fascia are incised to expose the tail of the breast.

Figure 12.81
Both pectoralis muscles are retracted to provide access to the axilla. Here, the tail of Spence and the low (level I) axillary nodes are removed (arrow).

Drainage and closure of the wound proceed as described in "Modified Radical Mastectomy" (next subsection).

MODIFIED RADICAL MASTECTOMY

A modified radical mastectomy (Patey operation) removes the breast, the fascia of the pectoralis major muscle, the pectoralis minor muscle, and all the axillary lymph nodes. By contrast, the Handley modified radical mastectomy spares the pectoralis minor muscle. Excision of the pectoralis minor muscle facilitates

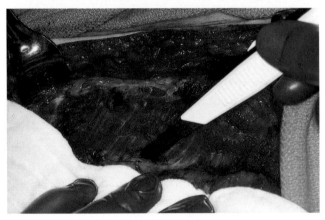

FIGURE 12.79

A few perforator blood vessels will be encountered near the sternum. Small vessels can be safely cauterized, but large ones should be ligated.

The dissection continues laterally toward the lateral border of the pectoralis major muscle.

Figure 12.80
The lateral border of the pectoralis major muscle is now dissected along its entire length, from the axilla (superiorly) to its costal insertion (inferiorly).

At this point, the breast has been completely detached from the muscle. It is now reflected laterally,

a more thorough axillary dissection. When a complete axillary node dissection is indicated, the Patey operation is the procedure of choice.

The indications for a modified radical mastectomy are

- large malignant tumors.
- microscopic, multifocal, and multicentric infiltrating cancer.
- malignant lesions with multiple ipsilateral primaries.
- diffuse malignant calcifications diagnosed on mammography.
- radiotherapy unavailable to the patient owing to patient's distance from the facility.

Surgical Technique – Modified Radical Mastectomy

PREPARATION

The skin of the anterior thorax, axilla, neck, arm, and upper abdomen is prepared with an antiseptic solution, and the area is draped. The area of the dissection is mapped.

The initial steps for a modified radical mastectomy are essentially the same as for a total mastectomy – that is, skin incision, dissection of the skin flaps, and dissection of the breast away from the pectoralis major muscle. For details, see "Total Mastectomy," Figures 12.66 through 12.79 (preceding subsection). The present description of the modified radical mastectomy begins at the point where dissection of the breast has reached the lateral border of the pectoralis major muscle (see Figure 12.80 in the preceding subsection).

Figure 12.82
The upper and lower skin flaps have been elevated off the breast and the breast has been dissected away from the pectoralis major muscle. The deep layer of the superficial fascia (arrow) is now incised along the lateral border of the pectoralis major muscle, and the muscle is skeletonized to free its lateral border.

Figure 12.83
When skeletonization is complete, the pectoralis major muscle is retracted upward and medially to expose the pectoralis minor muscle. The deep layer of the superficial fascia (arrow) is found below the undersurface of the pectoralis major.

Figure 12.84
The interpectoral lymph nodes are located between the pectoralis major and minor muscles. The location of the nodes on the posterior surface of the pectoralis major is just medial to the acromiothoracic

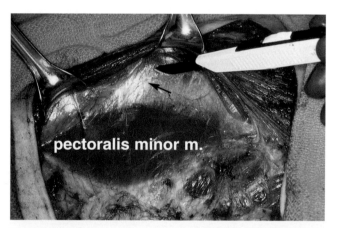

FIGURE 12.83

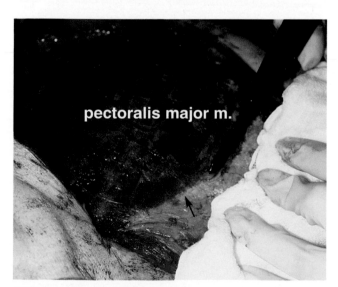

FIGURE 12.82

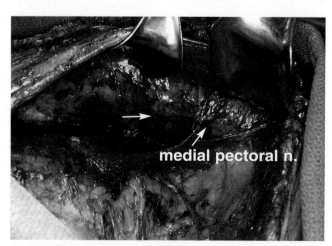

FIGURE 12.84

vessels and the lateral pectoral nerve – the so-called neurovascular bundle to the pectoralis major muscle (arrow) – and *not* along the superior surface of the pectoralis minor muscle.

Figure 12.85

When the clinical indication is to excise the interpectoral lymph nodes, the deep layer of the superficial pectoralis fascia is excised. That dissection must be carefully done to avoid injury to the lateral pectoral nerve. Severing that nerve results in atrophy of the sternal insertion portion of the pectoralis major muscle (arrow).

Figure 12.86

The pectoralis major muscle is being retracted upward and medially. The pectoralis minor muscle is skeletonized on its medial and lateral borders. Vascular clips or sutures are placed above and below the borders to mark the axillary levels.

Figure 12.87

The surgeon uses the index and middle fingers of the non-dominant hand (blunt dissection) to dissect the posterior surface of the pectoralis minor muscle away from the chest wall.

Branches of the lateral and medial pectoral nerves are quite intimate to the pectoralis minor

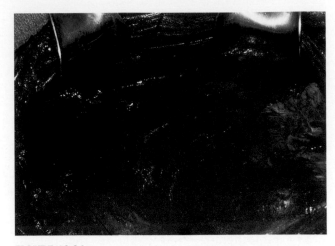

FIGURE 12.86

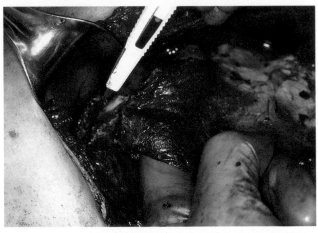

FIGURE 12.87

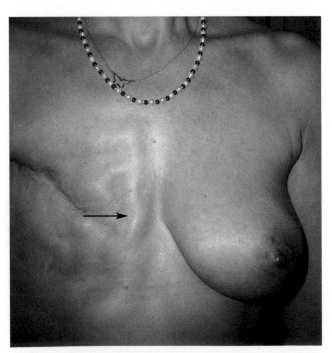

FIGURE 12.85

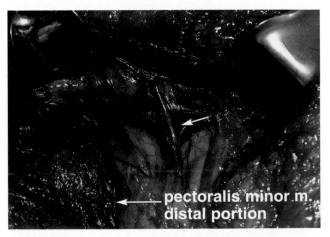

FIGURE 12.88

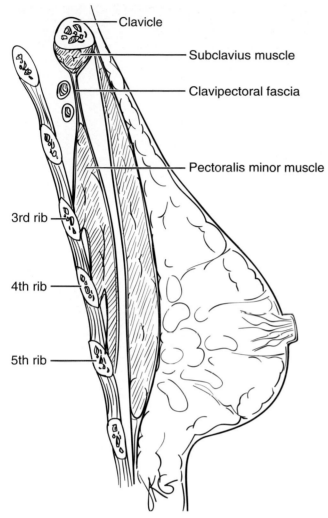

- Clavicle
- Subclavius muscle
- Clavipectoral fascia
- Pectoralis minor muscle

3rd rib
4th rib
5th rib

FIGURE 12.89

muscle. During skeletonization, care should be taken to avoid injury to those nerves. Dissection of the posterior surface of the muscle should commence at the upper third of the muscle. The surgeon must keep his or her fingers parallel to the clavicle to avoid injury to the axillary vein.

Figure 12.88

Having taken the appropriate precautions, the surgeon now transects the insertion of the pectoralis minor muscle near its insertion in the coracoid process and distal to the medial pectoral nerve where that nerve loops around the muscle (arrow). Because this portion of the pectoralis minor muscle contains no major blood vessels, hemostasis uses electrocautery rather than clamping of individual blood vessels.

Figure 12.88 demonstrates the transection of the pectoralis minor distal to the medial pectoral

nerve. The proximal end of the severed muscle has retracted; it is proximal and behind the nerve. At this point, the retracted distal portion of the muscle remains attached to its origin in the ribs. The muscle will be removed after the axillary dissection is complete.

Figures 12.89 and 12.90

The next step in the operation is to transect the clavipectoral fascia to expose the axillary vein and the axillary contents (Figure 12.90).

A drawing (Figure 12.89) shows the relationships among the clavipectoral fascia, the pectoralis minor muscle, and the axillary vessels. Superiorly, at the level of the first and second ribs, the clavipectoral fascia coalesces with the costocoracoid membrane to envelop the subclavius muscle and become the ligament of Halsted medialy. That ligament is the most apical anatomic structure of the axilla and an anatomic landmark during dissection of all three levels of the axillary lymph nodes.

Figure 12.91

The initial step of the axillary node dissection is to find the axillary vein (arrow), which is easily distinguished from the surrounding fat by its contrasting blue color.

Dissection of the axilla commences near the tendinous portion of the latissimus dorsi muscle laterally and continues medially toward the apex of the axilla. The dissection along the inferior border of the axillary vein should be done gently, leaving the adventitia. Arm edema is minimized when trauma to the axillary vein is avoided.

Four tributaries are encountered as the axillary vein is dissected medially. Medial to lateral, they are

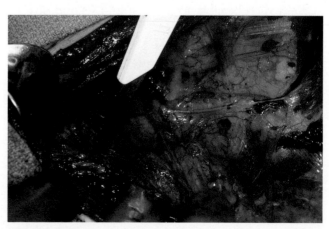

FIGURE 12.90

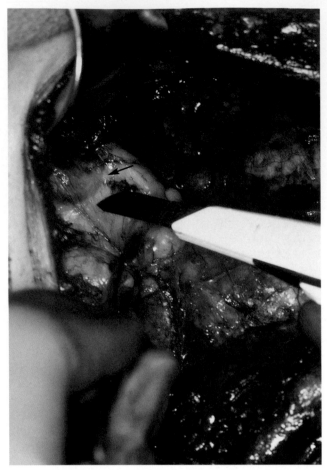

FIGURE 12.91

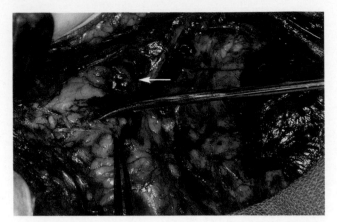

FIGURE 12.92

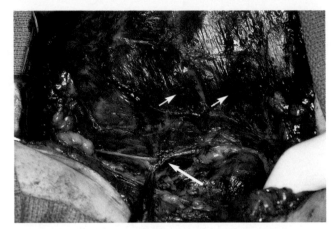

FIGURE 12.93

the thoracic, the pectoral, the lateral thoracic, and the dorsal thoracic veins. Each must be transected between ligatures.

Figure 12.92
Dissection continues toward the apex to find the ligament of Halsted (arrow) and the costocoracoid fascia, which lie close to the first and second ribs.

Figures 12.93 and 12.94
As the dissection continues, two nerves – the long thoracic and the thoracodorsal – should be identified. The long thoracic nerve is the most medial of the two. As it emerges in the chest, it continues as a single trunk to the level of the third rib. At that point, it starts to give branches that innervate the fascicles of the serratus anterior muscle (small arrows).

To prevent injury to any of those branches, the long thoracic nerve should be identified where it makes its appearance on the chest. The nerve is not close to the chest wall. On its downward course

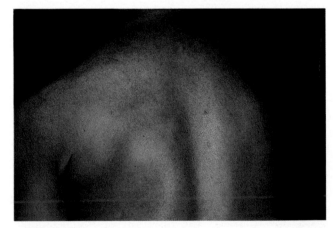

FIGURE 12.94

along the thoracic wall, it runs within the fascia of the serratus anterior muscle. The fascia of the serratus anterior must be divided (large arrow) so that the nerve can be isolated.

Stimulation of the nerve with a forceps or clamp causes postoperative paresthesia (possibly very trouble-

some) and should be avoided. Severance of the long thoracic nerve causes paralysis of the serratus anterior muscle, resulting in a "winged" scapula (Figure 12.94).

Figure 12.95
Now the thoracodorsal nerve must be identified. Figure 12.95 demonstrates, in a right mastectomy, the subscapularis vein as it enters the axillary vein (arrow A). The subscapularis vein is a landmark for finding the thoracodorsal nerve (arrow B), which is always located medial to the vein.

Figure 12.96
With both nerves – the long thoracic and the thoracodorsal – under vision, the axillary fat pad that lies between them is dissected by sharp dissection using scissors. The scissors is kept slightly open while "pushing" the fat down. Dissection continues downward to where the distal portion of the pectoralis minor muscle (transected earlier in the dissection) is still attached to its insertion on the ribs (arrow).

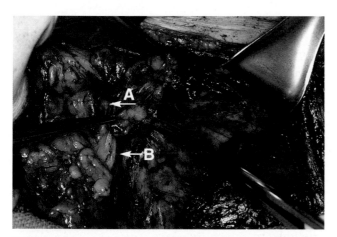

FIGURE 12.95

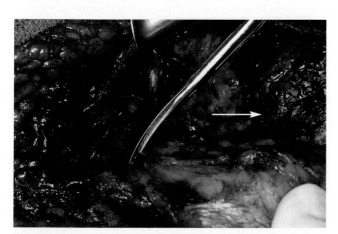

FIGURE 12.96

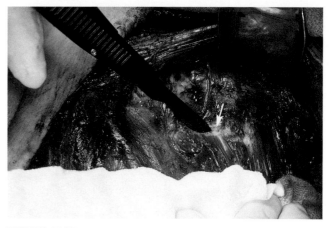

FIGURE 12.97

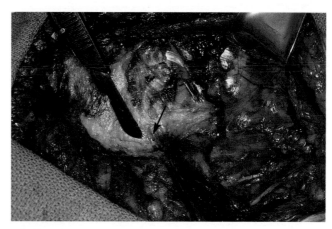

FIGURE 12.98

Figures 12.97 and 12.98
The distal end of the pectoralis minor muscle is excised from its insertion on the third, fourth, and fifth ribs by sharp dissection along the fascia that separates the pectoralis minor from the serratus muscles (arrows).

Figure 12.99
In the same anatomic plane, dissection continues down in the direction of the latissimus dorsi muscle, at which point the pectoralis minor is completely detached from the chest wall and becomes incorporated to the specimen.

Figure 12.100
Figure 12.100 shows the axilla upon completion of the axillary dissection. The long thoracic nerve is seen lying over the serratus anterior muscle. The thoracodorsal nerve crosses medial-to-lateral over the subscapularis vein and enters the latissimus dorsi muscle along its medial surface.

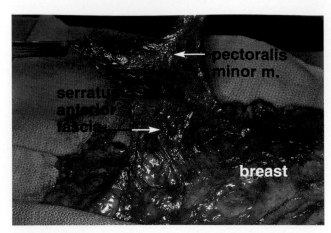

FIGURE 12.99

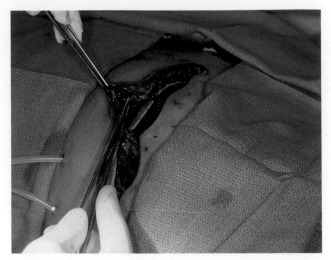

FIGURE 12.101A

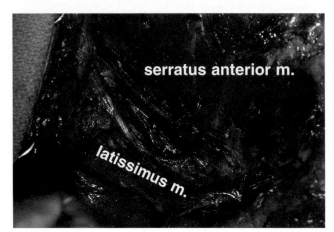

FIGURE 12.100

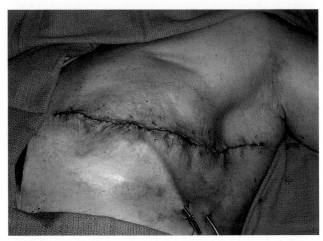

FIGURE 12.101B

If large metastatic nodes are present along the course of the thoracodorsal nerve, that nerve can be sacrificed for a more thorough node dissection. The disability that results from severing the nerve causes internal rotation of the arm, but doses not disturb arm function.

CLOSURE

After hemostasis is secured, the wound is irrigated with lukewarm water. Water should be used rather than saline solution, because osmolarity will cause floating cells in the operative field to break down. They can then be suctioned out with the irrigation.

Excess skin from the skin flaps should be trimmed to produce a more cosmetically acceptable scar.

Figure 12.101A and 12.101B

Two close suction catheters – one for the upper skin flap and one for the lower – are placed in the wound. They are brought out through separate stub wounds made in the lower skin flap and are secured

to the skin with sutures. The drains will be connected to a negative-pressure device. They stay in for approximately four to five days.

The subcutaneous tissue layer is approximated with interrupted sutures of 2/0 plain catgut (A). The skin is approximated with a continuous subcuticular stitch, using monofilament absorbable suture material (B).

A pressure dressing should be applied to keep the skin flaps close to the chest wall.

Figure 12.102

Postoperatively, the lateral half of a modified radical mastectomy scar is hidden under the pectoralis major muscle.

COMPLICATIONS

Postoperative loss of sensation on the anterior chest wall and the inner surface of the ipsilateral

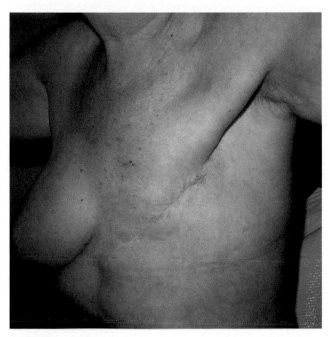

FIGURE 12.102

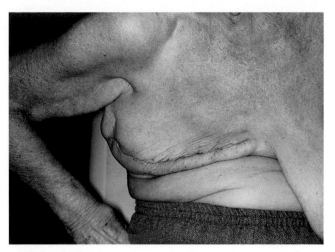

FIGURE 12.103A

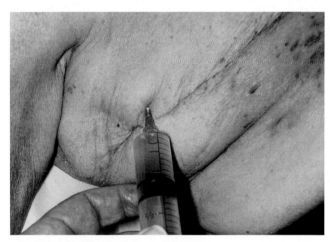

FIGURE 12.103B

arm is a common occurrence with a modified radical mastectomy. The severing of the sensory nerve branches of the lateral and anterior cutaneous nerves of the second through the sixth intercostal nerves and of the intercostobrachial nerves produce this loss of sensation, which is not considered a complication.

Complications that may follow a total mastectomy or modified radical mastectomy are

- wound infection,
- bleeding,
- seroma,
- skin slough,
- nerve injury, and
- lymphedema of the arm.

Postoperative **wound infection** and **bleeding** can be prevented by careful surgical technique and by proper hemostasis during dissection of the skin flaps.

Figure 12.103A and 12.103B

Seroma is one of the most common complications following a modified radical mastectomy (A). It occurs more frequently in obese patients. To prevent this complication, the drains should remain in place for a longer period.

Small seromas are treated using aspiration (B). Large, recurrent seromas should be incised and drained.

Figure 12.104A and 12.104B

A truly dreadful complication of modified radical mastectomy is **sloughing (necrosis) of the skin flaps** (A). Viable skin flaps can always be obtained if dissected evenly and in the proper tissue plane, with a thin layer of subcutaneous tissue left attached. Careful dissection of the flaps and tensionless closure can prevent this complication. Unless the area of the slough is extensive, the complication can be resolved with local debridement and frequent skin cleansing (B).

The adverse effects of the **injury to the nerves** (pectoral, thoracodorsal, long thoracic) were already discussed in "Applied Surgical Anatomy of the Breast" earlier in this chapter. Again, briefly, injury to the medial pectoral nerve causes atrophy in the clavicular portion of the pectoralis major muscle. Injury to the lateral pectoral nerve causes atrophy in the sternal and abdominal portions of the same muscle. Injury to the thoracodorsal nerve results in impair-

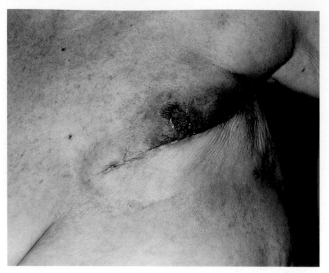

FIGURE 12.104A

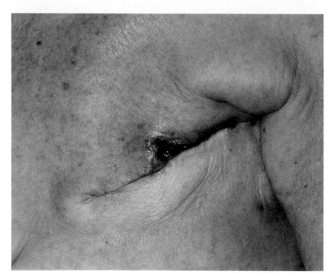

FIGURE 12.104B

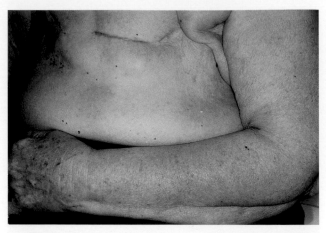

FIGURE 12.105

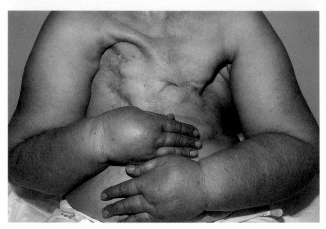

FIGURE 12.106

ment to external rotation of the ipsilateral arm. Injury to the long thoracic nerve causes a "winged" scapula, which is the most disabling and cosmetically unacceptable of the nerve complications.

Transient swelling of the arm is not uncommon following a modified radical mastectomy. **Lymphedema of the arm** is preventable. The complication is related not to the number of nodes removed, but to the axillary vein being subjected to trauma during the axillary dissection. To avoid or to minimize the complication, dissection of the axillary vein should be gentle and should leave the adventitia attached to the vein. If a phlebotomy or intravenous injection must be given on the ipsilateral arm, the skin should be thoroughly cleansed to avoid inflammation or infection.

Figure 12.105
Occasionally, lymphedema of the arm may be complicated by cellulitis of the skin. The arm becomes hard in a clinical presentation called "brawny lymphedema."

In the acute phase, brawny lymphedema should be treated with antibiotics and elevation of the arm.

Figure 12.106
When the cellulitis subsides, the patient should wear a pressure-gradient elastic sleeve.

Marked edema of the arm was more common when radical mastectomy was the only treatment for breast cancer. Fortunately, the more conservative surgical procedures of today make lymphedema largely anecdotal.

RADICAL MASTECTOMY

In the 1960s, radical mastectomy was the only surgical therapy available to treat breast cancer. Today,

with early detection and use of adjuvant therapy to downstage the disease, the procedure is seldom indicated. The only indications still current are

- tumor fixed to the fascia or pectoralis muscle, and
- metastases to the interpectoral nodes.

Even when a radical mastectomy is indicated, the procedure used today is not the classic radical mastectomy originally described by Halsted (excision of the pectoralis major muscle close to its clavicular and sternal origin). Because the breast parenchyma extends only to the level of the second rib and to the lateral border of the sternum, excising the portion of the pectoralis major muscle attached to those bony structures is unnecessary. Preserving them gives the patient a more cosmetically acceptable postoperative appearance.

Figures 12.107 through 12.110 illustrate the evolution of the radical mastectomy.

Figure 12.107

The right radical mastectomy shown in Figure 12.107 was done in the late 1960s. Excision of the pectoralis major muscle included the clavicular and sternal origins of that muscle. The vertical incision in common use at that time restricted the patient's summer wardrobe choices.

Figure 12.108

The right radical mastectomy shown in Figure 12.108 done in the late 1970s. The clavicular and ster-

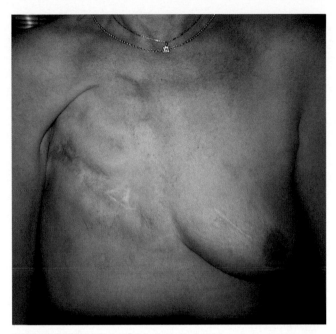

FIGURE 12.108

nal origins of the pectoralis major muscle were spared, and a transverse mastectomy incision was used. The postoperative cosmetic appearance is more acceptable.

Figure 12.109

The radical mastectomy shown in Figure 12.109 was done in the late 1980s. The lesion was located in the upper middle quadrant of the breast and was attached to the pectoralis major muscle. The patient received three preoperative cycles of chemotherapy to downstage the disease. The transverse incision commenced at the anterior border of the latissimus dorsi muscle, continued transversely to the middle of the chest, and then extended vertically downward to in-

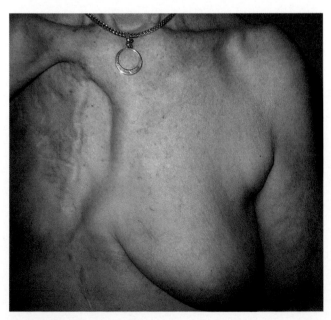

FIGURE 12.107

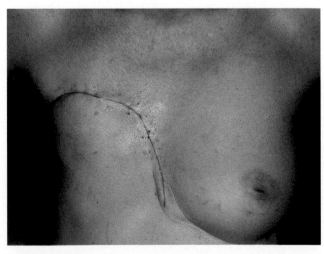

FIGURE 12.109

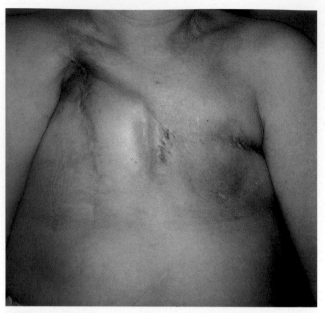

FIGURE 12.110

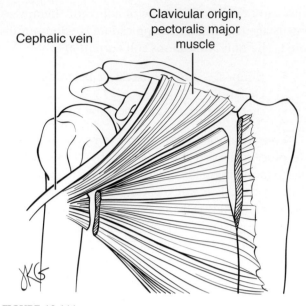

FIGURE 12.111

clude the areola and the nipple. The clavicular and sternal origins of the pectoralis muscles were spared. Chemotherapy was continued for six more cycles after the surgery.

Figure 12.110

The right radical mastectomy shown in Figure 12.110 was done in the early 1960s. The clavicular portion of the pectoralis major muscle was excised very close to its origin in the clavicle. That excision and the vertical incision contributed to an undesirable cosmetic result. The patient underwent a left total mastectomy 12 years later for advanced metachronous breast cancer.

Surgical Technique – Radical Mastectomy

PREPARATION

A radical mastectomy requires general anesthesia.

The incision and the extent of the skin flaps are mapped onto the skin. When possible, a transverse or slightly oblique incision is preferable.

INCISION

The surgical technique for the incision and the dissection of the skin flaps is essentially the same as for a total mastectomy (see "Surgical Technique – Total Mastectomy," Figures 12.73 through 12.78). The only difference is that, for a radical mastectomy, the dissection of the upper skin flap is carried past

the clavicle, exposing the cephalic vein that separates the deltoid muscle from the pectoralis major.

Figure 12.111

The clavicular origin of the pectoralis major muscle is spared. To separate the clavicular origin from the sternal origin, the fascia of the muscle is incised. Then, the surgeon uses the blunt side of a dissecting scissors and the index finger of the non-dominant hand to separate the muscle fibers. Through the resulting opening, the muscle fibers are separated from medial to lateral.

The lateral portion ends close to the insertion into the humerus. There, the tendinous portion of the muscle is skeletonized and transected as the surgeon uses the index finger of the non-dominant hand to retract it upward and laterally. The clavicular portion of the muscle is spared. Small blood vessels are clamped and tied as they are encountered.

EXCISION

Figure 12.112

As the sternal origin of the muscle is approached, the surgeon introduces the index finger of the non-dominant hand into the plane between the pectoralis major muscle and the thoracic wall. The pectoralis muscle is lifted using the index finger and thumb, and the muscle is cut serially in the direction of its abdominal insertion. A rim of muscle approximately 1–2 cm in size is left attached to the sternum.

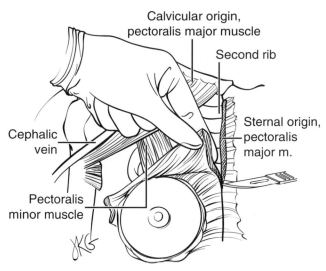

FIGURE 12.112

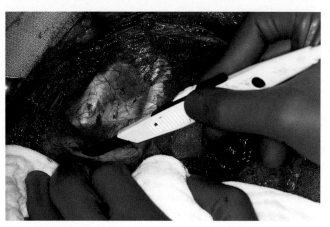

FIGURE 12.113

The perforating branches of the internal mammary artery are clamped, transected, and ligated as they are encountered during the dissection.

Figure 12.113

When the transection is complete, the muscle is detached from the chest wall starting medially near the sternum and proceeding laterally in a tissue plane between the fascia and the chest wall. Dissection continues until the pectoralis minor muscle is exposed.

Excision of the pectoralis minor muscle facilitates the axillary dissection. The pectoralis minor muscle is skeletonized and transected near its insertion on the coracoid process. The origins of the muscle on the third, fourth, and fifth ribs are temporarily left attached to the ribs. The muscle will be excised and incorporated into the specimen once the axillary dissection is complete.

The surgical technique for the axillary node dissection of a radical mastectomy does not differ from the one done in a modified radical mastectomy. The reader should refer to Figures 12.89 through 12.100 when reading the following paragraphs.

The clavipectoral fascia is incised, the axilla is entered, and the axillary vein is exposed. A medial-to-lateral dissection of the axilla commences laterally at the ligament of Halsted. Once the ligament has been transected, a tie is placed on the distal por-

tion of the cut end of the specimen to situate it for the pathologist.

Tributary branches of the axillary vein are divided between clamps and ligated. Medial to lateral, those branches are the thoracic, the pectoral, the lateral thoracic, and the dorsal thoracic veins.

The nerves to the latissimus dorsi and serratus anterior muscles will be seen during the dissection. The more medial nerve, the long thoracic, is dissected away from the axillary fascia and spared. The more lateral nerve, the thoracodorsal, innervates the latissimus dorsi. That nerve can be sacrificed if the adjacent nodes are grossly involved with metastasis. The disability caused by severing the nerve is minimal.

Dissection of the axilla continues down to the origin of the pectoralis minor muscle on the third, fourth, and fifth ribs. At that level, the muscle is transected. The muscle is thereby incorporated into the specimen. Dissection then continues toward the anterior border of the latissimus dorsi muscle, at which point the breast is removed.

CLOSURE

The previously described closure techniques are applied, and the area of the dissection is drained to negative suction.

COMPLICATIONS

The complications following a radical mastectomy are similar to those described for a modified radical mastectomy. The incidence of lymphedema is greater following a radical mastectomy.

13

Role of the Plastic Surgeon

NORMAN H. SCHULMAN, MD FACS

Post-mastectomy breast reconstruction is a major component of the practice of plastic and reconstructive surgery. It offers women who must undergo a mastectomy options for restoring the female contour and appearance.

Breast reconstruction is a readily performed procedure that yields pleasing results for practically all women requiring mastectomy. A reconstruction can immediately follow a mastectomy procedure, or it may be done at a later time. The available techniques are many and varied. Selection of a technique depends on a thorough understanding of goals, alternatives, and risks by the patient and the physician alike. No single reconstruction technique is ideal for all patients, and the role played by the oncology surgeon significantly affects the ultimate selection of surgical reconstruction. The plastic surgeon must consider each of those factors when counseling a patient.

This chapter outlines the main aspects of breast and nipple – areola reconstruction. Its purpose is to guide the practitioner in counseling patients who have made a decision for surgical breast cancer treatment and breast reconstruction.

TIMING

Breast reconstruction can be immediate or delayed.

Immediate Reconstruction

Immediate breast reconstruction holds two main advantages for the patient:

- Tissue planes are more malleable when freshly dissected. Scarring has not yet developed, and the tissue is more elastic and flexible. Landmarks and anatomy are not distorted.

- An emotional advantage is gained. The "loss of a body part" grief syndrome is attenuated by the immediate reconstruction.

Disadvantages must also be considered, however. The two mentioned here are rare, but should be explained to the patient beforehand:

- The plan may be to use a prosthesis or tissue expander; but, if local muscle has to be sacrificed during the mastectomy dissection, or if it is very poorly developed, adequately protecting a prosthesis or expander is more difficult.
- If radiation unexpectedly follows primary care, the reconstruction may be compromised.

The advantages far outweigh the disadvantages. The reconstruction procedure is significantly easier at the time of mastectomy because of the fresh tissue condition. The emotional gain is also significant. At the present time, criteria for radiation includes a finding of three or more positive lymph nodes. That finding may not be apparent until the final pathology report, after the reconstruction has been completed. Radiation has the potential for complicating reconstruction, but techniques are available to minimize the effect without compromising tumor therapy.

Delayed Reconstruction

The advantages of delayed reconstruction are tied chiefly to the greater information then available about pathology findings and about adjuvant therapy:

- The final histopathology report is available, including the findings concerning metastatic lymph nodes (if any).
- Adjuvant therapy is complete.

Disadvantages are both physical and psychological:

- The woman undergoes another surgical procedure, with its concomitant risks, including anesthesia.
- Before reconstruction can occur, the woman may go through the emotional trauma associated with observed loss of a body part.

From a clinical viewpoint, the reasons to delay reconstruction are few and not compelling. However, if the tumor is extensive, and radiation therapy is known to be required as part of the primary modality, then delayed reconstruction is preferable.

TECHNIQUES

The techniques used in a breast reconstruction may be prosthetic or autogenous. Prosthetic devices are those fabricated by medical supply companies – breast implants, for example. Autogenous sources are those supplied by the patient – skin or fat transferred from other body sites.

Prosthetic Reconstruction

Reconstruction using prosthetic devices has the advantage of shorter additional operating time after the mastectomy. Also, no additional incisions (with accompanying scarring) are made.

In terms of disadvantages, all prosthetics (not just breast implants) sometimes fail. Failure of a long-term prosthetic device necessitates further surgery. Also, as a patient ages, a prosthesis may no longer match the other breast.

HISTORY

Prosthetic reconstruction involves placement of devices into the body under the skin and muscles of the chest wall. The devices simulate the appearance and "feel" of a normal breast. They are balloons fabricated from silicone polymers and filled with saline or silicone gel or a combination of both.

Silicone implants were first used in 1962 after a great deal of research conducted in the 1940s and 1950s showed that silicone implants could be used for cosmetic enhancement of otherwise normal breasts. In the late 1960s, the devices were placed under the scarred, contracted skin of patients who had undergone previous mastectomies. These early reconstructions were devised to help patients by precluding the need for them to place a rubber prosthesis into a brassiere. This method of simulating a normal breast under clothing had been a difficult and embarrassing procedure for many women.

The early reconstruction efforts were not particularly aesthetically pleasing. Not until the 1970s – when techniques for replacing the missing skin envelope came into use – were prosthetic breast reconstructions seen as aesthetically desirable.

Before that time, radical mastectomy, a procedure that sacrifices the pectoralis major muscle (leaving a severe chest wall deformity), was the most common form of mastectomy. Modified radical mastectomy, a procedure that spares the pectoralis major muscle (and is just as effective a cancer treatment in practically all cases), provided a much more amenable background for reconstruction. If adequate tissue remained, then an appropriately sized implant placed under the remaining skin and muscle would result in an acceptable replacement of contour. However, most patients lacked the necessary surplus tissue, and techniques were sought to replace the skin lost with the mastectomy.

The use of local tissue or flaps was often quite successful, but the surgery was more extensive and additional scarring resulted. In 1983, Radovan introduced a stretching device ("expander"), which has since become the surgical standard for prosthetic reconstruction.

THE EXPANDER TECHNIQUE

Figure 13.1
Preoperative (A). A balloon made of silicone polymer is inserted under the remaining tissues after the mastectomy on the chest wall – usually the pectoralis major and serratus anterior muscles. The balloon is not permanent; it is designed only to stretch the skin so that the desired restoration can be achieved. The balloon includes a filling valve. At the initial reconstruction surgery, just enough saline solution is injected into the balloon to allow tension-free closure of the patient's remaining skin.

The balloon comes in various sizes. The size selected for a particular reconstruction depends on the size of the specimen and the size of the opposite breast, or (in the case of a double mastectomy) the desired final size of the reconstructed breasts and the ability of the patient's form to accommodate a particular size.

After an average of two weeks for wound healing, the balloon begins to be progressively inflated.

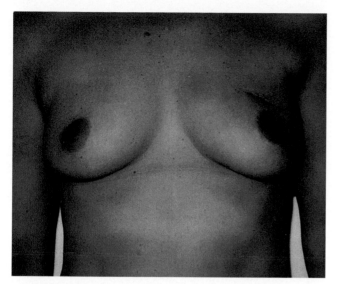

FIGURE 13.1A

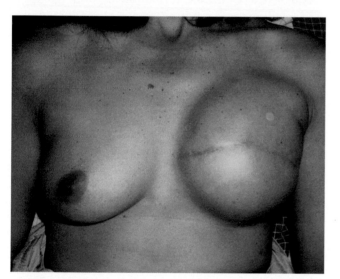

FIGURE 13.1B

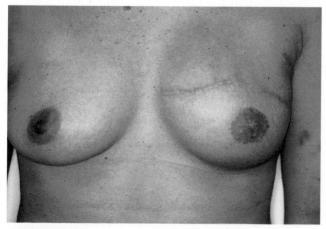

FIGURE 13.1C

Inflation is usually incremented weekly by an injection of between 40 mL and 100 mL of additional saline into the balloon. The quantity depends on the patient's comfort and the ability of her skin to stretch. The increased pressure from the weekly inflation increment usually subsides within 72 hours.

It usually takes between three and six weeks to fully stretch the balloon. Over-stretching by about 20%–30% is encouraged. The extra space allows for eventual shrinkage and provides a natural droop (ptosis) once the permanent prosthesis is inserted (B).

The balloon is usually left in place for at least four months to allow for tissue accommodation and to minimize "memory loss" shrinkage. An expander may be left in place until adjuvant chemotherapy (if required) is complete. That period averages six months; in some cases, it is slightly longer. Most tissue expanders can be safely left in place for about one year. They must be replaced by that time because, with a few exceptions ("permanent expanders" or "adjustable implants"), expanders are not made for sustained use.

When the time comes for removal of the expander, the patient returns to the hospital, either as an outpatient or for a one-night stay, and the expander is replaced by an implant designed for long-term use. At the time of this second procedure, ancillary procedures may also be performed:

- Adjusting the expander pocket to obtain the correct height for the permanent implant
- Redefining the inframammary crease to create a realistic look (especially a natural amount of breast droop)
- Adjusting a remaining normal breast by reduction, elevation, or (less frequently) augmentation to better match the reconstructed breast

Nipple–areola reconstruction is usually performed at this second stage, although some surgeons choose to perform nipple–areola reconstruction at a third stage (often as an office procedure), if the most desirable nipple–areola location is difficult to determine at the time of expander removal.

The technique of tissue expansion, commonly performed at the time of the mastectomy and followed by later placement of a permanent breast implant with tissue adjustment and nipple–areola reconstruction, is the most common form of post-mastectomy reconstruction performed in the United States today (C).

CURRENTLY AVAILABLE IMPLANTS

Permanent breast implants may consist of

- saline-filled balloons whose walls are made of silicone polymers ("saline implant").
- silicone-filled balloons whose walls are made from silicone polymers ("silicone-gel implant").
- a nested pair of balloons, the outer balloon usually containing silicone, and the inner one, saline ("combination implant").

Each of these implant types has its own advantages and disadvantages.

On the plus side, **saline implants** usually have a fill range (10–40 mL variance) that allows for adjustment. (The implant is softer if filled to the lower end of the manufacturer's suggested fill range.) A saline implant may be easier to remove and replace after long-term use. On the other hand, saline implants usually do not feel "natural." They may be too hard if over-filled. If the implant is filled only to manufacturer's minimum requirement, "ripples" may appear if the patient's overlying skin and muscle layers are thin.

Saline implants have an ultimate failure rate of between 6% and 8%. (The filler valve may eventually fail, or the balloon may wear out from abnormal rubbing of creases.)

Silicone-gel implants provide a more natural form and shape. If skin and muscle coverage is thin, they show little or no rippling, and a more natural reconstruction is easier to achieve, particularly in terms of matching a remaining normal breast. Silicone-gel implants have a low failure rate; they have remained in place in many patients for more than 30 years. Nevertheless, at the present time, the U.S. Food and Drug Administration will allow the use of silicone-gel implants in reconstructions only if saline is deemed inappropriate (for example, in a situation of very thin overlying skin and muscle, or previous failure or unsatisfactory result with a saline device). All recipients of silicone-gel devices must enter a government-sponsored follow-up program and agree to the conditions outlined in a lengthy consent form containing multiple disclaimers.

If a silicone-gel implant fails, the cause is most often trauma. Traumatic failure can cause the gel contents not only to leave the balloon, but to break out of the body's own protective capsule. (The body forms scar tissue called a "capsule" around any implanted device.) Trauma of this kind can result in painful scar tissue that must be removed, sometimes

with difficulty. A magnetic resonance imaging (MRI) exam may be required to confirm the implant failure.

Combination implants combine all the best qualities of silicone and saline. They can be adjusted to a finer degree, even after surgery. However, they cost considerably more than standard saline or silicone-gel implants, and they are subject to same risks of failure as the other implants – especially faulty valves on the saline component.

Selection of a particular breast implant requires a lengthy and detailed discussion between the patient and her surgeon. The various devices, their advantages and disadvantages, and their characteristics all have to be fully weighed and balanced against the patient's goals, the best achievable result, and the patient's clinical condition and comfort.

No prosthetic breast implant is perfect. All may produce heavy capsule formation or undergo traumatic failure, necessitating re-operation for adjustment or replacement. However, these subsequent surgeries are usually minor outpatient procedures.

Autogenous Reconstruction

Reconstruction using the patient's own tissues has the advantage of producing pleasing, natural-looking results. Moreover, after the initial healing and any final adjustments, further surgery is almost never required. However, this type of reconstruction surgery is more prone to medical complications because of the additional tissue manipulation and longer operating time. Additional surgical sites mean additional scarring, and convalescence takes considerably longer.

THE AUTOGENOUS TECHNIQUE

The autogenous technique takes tissue from an area other than the breast and moves it into the site of the removed breast. Tissue moved in this manner is called a "flap." The term "flap" implies a "stalk." The stalk must provide oxygenating and nourishing components – arteries and veins.

Flaps are classified into two categories:

- Pedicled flaps maintain their primary vascular attachment in the form of a stalk.
- "Free" flaps are detached from their primary blood supply and reattached by microsurgical techniques at the chest wall site.

Flaps are the ideal method of reconstruction. Because flaps contain only native tissue, they gain and lose weight with the patient. Once the surgical reconstruction and adjustment for size have been

completed, re-operation is rarely required. However, the availability and use of a flap is highly dependent on certain factors related to the patient: availability of tissue, previous surgical history, history of smoking, and overall medical condition.

Common pedicled flaps include the latissimus dorsi flap and the transrectus abdominal muscle (TRAM) flap. Free flaps can come from the TRAM or latissimus regions, or from the upper or lower gluteal areas of the buttocks.

PEDICLED FLAPS

Figure 13.2
The **latissimus dorsi flap** contains skin, fat, and muscle from the back (pre-operative view [A]). The flap is passed through the axilla onto the surface of the chest wall at the mastectomy site. The flap keeps its own blood supply, the thoracodorsal blood vessels, which are long enough to reach the chest site. The subcutaneous tissues and skin are sutured into the defect left by the removed breast (B).

The latissimus dorsi flap is a hearty flap that can be used in almost all clinical situations (smoking, diabetes, prior irradiation). Its blood supply is large, constant, and reliable. Often, however, the skin and fat on the back are not enough to simulate a breast unless an implant is also used. The surgery also requires closure at the donor site, which limits flap size and produces additional scarring on the back.

Figure 13.3
The **TRAM flap** contains skin, fat, and muscle from the lower abdominal wall (pre-operative view,

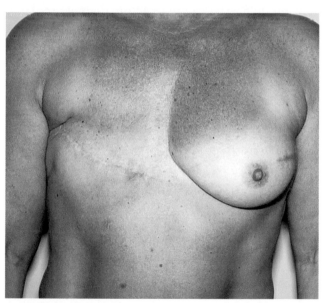

FIGURE 13.2A

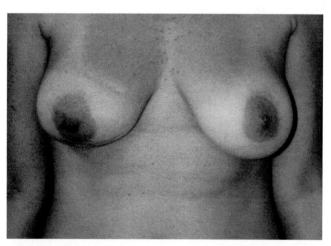

FIGURE 13.3A

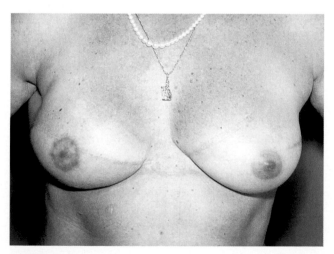

FIGURE 13.2B

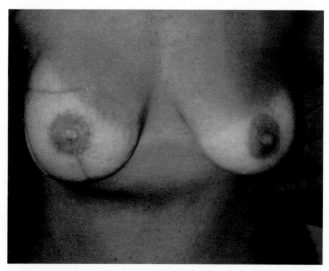

FIGURE 13.3B

right breast [A]). It is passed through a subcutaneous tunnel onto the surface of the chest wall at the mastectomy site (B). The flap is nourished by a blood vessel that courses through the rectus abdominal muscle (the internal mammary artery, which is renamed the superior epigastric artery once it enters the superior aspect of the rectus muscle).

The TRAM flap has many variants: ipsilateral or contralateral source, use of a single rectus muscle stalk or of both rectus muscles (for double reconstructions, or the building of a single large breast).

The TRAM flap usually provides more than enough tissue; a prosthesis is hardly ever required in conjunction with it. The completed reconstruction has a totally natural feel and appearance (B). Moreover, the donor site – the abdomen – becomes thinner owing to a simultaneous "tummy tuck." However, the procedure creates a large transabdominal scar, and the patient loses some function (that of the "borrowed" rectus muscle). Moreover, the vascularity of the flap is variable; survival of the entire flap is not assured. Spotty, hard areas of fat necrosis may appear. Also, the weakened abdominal wall may develop a bulge or hernia despite the most careful closure of the fascia, with or without mesh reinforcement.

The TRAM flap can only be used once. If the second breast must later be removed, this flap is no longer available. Double reconstructions must be carried out simultaneously or not at all.

Both pedicled flaps described here are versatile and, when appropriately used, may result in an excellent post-mastectomy reconstruction (2B) (3B).

The TRAM flap is the one most commonly used. The patient must have adequate but not excessive lower abdominal wall tissue. Obesity is a contraindication, because the fat may lack adequate circulation once elevated. Prior abdominal-wall surgery precludes the use of this flap, particularly if the superior epigastric blood supply has been interrupted on one or both sides. An exception to this rule occurs in the case of a transverse suprapubic incision, as used in most cesarean sections where only the lower portion of the blood supply is divided.) Prior liposuction of the abdominal wall is a direct contraindication, as is diabetes and a significant history of cigarette smoking. If part or all of the flap fails to survive, it is either trimmed, removed, or replaced with a latissimus dorsi flap (if that flap is available).

The latissimus dorsi flap is commonly used if the TRAM is not suitable. In cases in which radiation to the chest wall follows the mastectomy, the skin will not normally stretch with tissue expansion. If a TRAM is neither available nor desired, the latissimus flap is the best alternative, given the understanding that an implant is still required to complete the contour reconstruction. Occasionally, in patients with small breasts, the latissimus dorsi flap may be adequate for reconstruction without an implant.

FREE FLAPS

Free flaps are those that are totally disconnected from their source and then attached to the chest wall using microsurgery techniques. The most common source is the lower abdomen in the rectus territory (TRAM region). Other sources are the latissimus area and the upper or lower gluteal areas of the buttocks.

Because a direct vascular connection is made to the inferior epigastric vessels in this technique (a much larger and more direct blood supply than the superior epigastric vessels), factors such as smoking, prior surgery, and obesity are less of a consideration. Flap survivability also does not require a vascular delay. (Vascular delay [a technique to enhance survival of a pedicled TRAM flap] is a minor surgical procedure carried out two or three weeks before the main operation by clipping the inferior epigastric vessels.) Fewer complications such as partial flap loss and fat necrosis are seen.

But a free-flap procedure is also more difficult to perform than a pedicled TRAM. It requires microsurgery expertise and far more time under anesthesia in the operating room. Special microvascular monitoring equipment and personnel are also needed in the immediate postoperative period to insure vessel patency or to rescue microsurgical anastomoses if occlusion should occur.

PERFORATOR FREE FLAPS

Perforator free flaps are similar to free flaps, but only the blood vessels going to the fat and skin are used. Any muscle stalk is spared. These are taken primarily from the TRAM region, but with sparing of the rectus muscle.

The advantages with this type of flap are the same as with a TRAM flap, but the rectus muscle is spared. On the other hand, the dissection is long and tedious, and not universally successful. This technique also requires a high degree of specific microvascular surgical training.

Free flaps – either standard or perforator – produce the best reconstruction when transfer is successfully achieved. However, the procedures are reserved for use in large medical centers where microvascular surgery is performed, and trained staff

and equipment are on hand to insure success. Both procedures require significant additional anesthesia and operating room time – certainly an important criteria in patient selection.

Nipple–Areola Reconstruction

Nipple–areola reconstruction always uses the patient's own tissues and usually occurs as the final step in a reconstruction procedure. Medical tattooing may be used for all or part of the procedure.

Figure 13.4
Possible techniques for reconstructing the nipple–areola complex are

- tattooing an areola and nipple (darker shade) to simulate the nipple–areolar complex.
- sharing a nipple [composite graft from the opposite breast (A)].
- using a dermal-fat pedicle (B) for the nipple ("skate" flaps and modifications, star flaps, "Maltese cross", V-flaps).
- creating a full-thickness skin graft for the areola.

Many patients claim that they do not wish to have a reconstruction of the nipple–areola complex. However, once they see photographs of how well they look, and understand the safety and reliability of the procedure and its very low discomfort, they usually agree to this finishing touch. Reconstruction of the nipple–areola complex can be performed as the third and final phase of an expander reconstruction, but if the site is certain and adjustments minimal, it is often performed when the expander is exchanged for the permanent prosthesis.

In flap reconstruction – pedicled, free, or perforator – the procedure is performed at a second stage, when the flap is adjusted to match the opposite breast or vice versa. Occasionally, when placement is

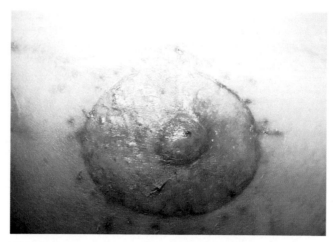

FIGURE 13.4A

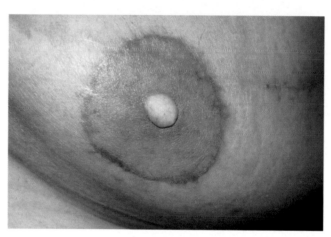

FIGURE 13.4B

uncertain at the second stage, reconstruction of the nipple–areola complex should be performed at a third stage no matter which technique is being used for breast reconstruction.

In summary; breast reconstruction may be offered to practically all women who must undergo mastectomy. It is generally a two or three staged procedure. The selection of, timing and technique must take into account all factors that may impact on the outcome and the patient's expectations.

Suggested Readings

GENERAL

Bland KI, Copeland EM, editors. 1991. The breast: comprehensive management of benign and malignant diseases. Philadelphia: Saunders.

Fitzpatrick TB. 1999. Fitzpatrick's dermatology in general medicine. New York: McGraw–Hill.

Haagensen CD. 1986. Diseases of the breast. 3rd ed. Philadelphia: Saunders.

Moore KL, Persaud TVN. 1998. The developing human: clinically oriented embryology. 6th ed. Philadelphia: Saunders.

FIBROADENOMA

Alle KM, Moss J, Venegas RJ, Khalkhali I, Klein SR. 1996. Conservative management of fibroadenoma of the breast. Br J Surg 83:992–3.

Dupont WD, Page DL, Parl FF, Vnencak-Jones CL, Plummer WD Jr, Rados MS, Schuyler PA. 1994. Long-term risk of breast cancer in women with fibroadenoma. N Engl J Med 331:10–15.

Hasson J, Pope CH. 1961. Mammary infarcts associated with pregnancy presenting as breast tumor. Surgery 49:331–46.

Levi F, Randimbison L, Te VC, La Vecchia C. 1994. Incidence of breast cancer in women with fibroadenoma. Int J Cancer 57:681–3.

Moran CS. 1935. Fibroadenoma of the breast during pregnancy and lactation. Arch Surg 31:688.

Noguchi S, Yokouchi H, Aihara T, Motomura K, Inaji H, Imaoka S, Koyama H. 1995. Progression of fibroadenoma to phyllodes tumor demonstrated by clonal analysis. Cancer 76:1779–85.

Recabaren JA Jr, Albano WA, Organ CH Jr. 1975. Giant adenofibroma of youth: a case report. Breast Dis 1:125.

Williamson ME, Lyons K, Hughes LE. 1993. Multiple fibroadenomas of the breast: a problem of uncertain incidence and management. Ann R Coll Surg Engl 75:161–3.

JUVENILE FIBROADENOMA

Mies C, Rosen PP. 1987. Juvenile fibroadenomas with atypical epithelial hyperplasia. Am J Surg Pathol 11:184–90.

HAMARTOMA

Abbitt PL, de Paredes ES, Sloop FB Jr. 1988. Breast hamartoma: a mammographic diagnosis. South Med J 81:167–70.

Hessler C, Schnyder P, Ozzello L. 1978. Hamartoma of the breast: diagnostic observation of 16 cases. Radiology 126:95–8.

PHYLLODES TUMOR

Al-Jurf A, Hawk WA, Crile G Jr. 1978. Cystosarcoma phyllodes. Surg Gynecol Obstet 46:358–64.

Ansah-Boateng Y, Tavassoll FA. 1992. Fibroadenoma and cystosarcoma phyllodes of the male breast. Mod Pathol 5:114–16.

Chua CL, Thomas A, Ng BK. 1989. Cystosarcoma phyllodes: a review of surgical options. 105:141–7.

Zurrida S, Bartoli C, Galimberti V, Squicciarini P, Delledonne V, Veronesi P, Bono A, de Palo G, Salvadori B. 1992. Which therapy for unexpected phyllode tumor of the breast? Eur J Cancer 28:654–7.

FIBROCYSTIC CHANGES

Minton JP. 1988. Dietary factors in benign breast disease. Cancer Bull 40:44.

Minton JP, Abou-Issa H. 1989. Nonendocrine theories of the etiology of benign breast disease. World J Surg 13:680–4.

Vorherr H. 1986. Fibrocystic breast disease: pathophysiology, pathomorphology, clinical picture, and management. Am J Obstet Gynecol 154:161–79.

Zylstra S. 1999. Office management of benign breast disease. Clin Obstet Gynecol 42:234–48.

CANCER

In Women

Ashikari R, Park K, Huvos AG, Urban JA. 1970. Paget's disease of the breast. Cancer 26:680–5.

Fisher B, Bryant J, Wolmark N, Mamounas E, Brown A, Fisher ER, Wickerham DL, Begovic M, DeCillis A, Robidoux A, and others. 1998. Effect of preoperative chemotherapy on the outcome of women with operable breast cancer. J Clin Oncol 6:2672–85.

Kister SJ, Haagensen CD. 1970. Paget's disease of the breast. Am J Surg 119:606–9.

Krecke KN, Gisvold JJ. 1993. Invasive lobular carcinoma of the breast: mammographic findings and extent of disease at diagnosis in 184 patients. AJR Am J Roentgenol 161:957–60.

Schwartz GF, Patchesfsky AS, Feig SA, Shaber GS, Schwartz AB. 1980. Multicentricity of non-palpable breast cancer. Cancer 45:2913–16.

Silverstein MJ, Waisman JR, Gamagami P, Gierson ED, Colburn WJ, Rosser RJ, Gordon PS, Lewinsky BS, Fingerhut A. 1990. Intraductal carcinoma of the breast (208 cases). Clinical factors influencing treatment choice. Cancer 66:102–8.

In Men

Crichlow RW. 1972. Carcinoma of the male breast. Surg Gynecol Obstet 134:1011–19.

Desai DC, Brennan EJ Jr, Carp NZ. 1996. Paget's disease of the male breast. Am Surg 62:1068–72.

Donegan WL. 1991. Cancer of the breast in men. CA Cancer J Clin 41:339–54.

Meyskens FL Jr, Tormey DC, Neifeld JP. 1976. Male breast cancer: a review. Cancer Treat Rev 3:83–93.

McLachlan SA, Erlichman C, Liu FF, Miller N, Pintilie M. 1996. Male breast cancer: an 11 year review of 66 patients. Breast Cancer Res Treat 40:225–30.

Sperlongano P, Pisaniello D. 2000. Current management of male abreast cancer. Ann Ital Chir 71:165–6.

Treves V. 1953. Inflammatory carcinoma of the breast in the male patient. Cancer 34:810.

NIPPLE DISCHARGE

Dixon JM, Scott WN, Miller WR. 1985. Natural history of cystic disease: the importance of cyst type. Br J Surg 72:190–2.

Leis HP Jr. 1961. The significance and treatment of nipple discharge. J Int Coll Surg 35:476.

Morrison C. 1998. The significance of nipple discharge: diagnosis and treatment regimes. Lippincotts Prim Care Pract 2:129–40.

Pilnik S, Leis HP Jr. 1978. Nipple discharge. In: Gallagher S, Leis HP Jr, Snyderman R, Urban J, editors. The breast. St. Louis: Mosby.

Urban JA. 1963. Excision of the major duct system of the breast. Cancer 16:516–20.

GYNECOMASTIA

Cavanaugh J, Niewoehner CB, Nuttall FQ. 1990. Gynecomastia and cirrhosis of the liver. Arch Intern Med 150:563–5.

Gruntmanis U, Braunstein GD. 2001. Treatment of gynecomastia. Curr Opin Investig Drugs 2:643–9.

Macmillan D, Nixon M. 2000. Gynecomastia: when is action required? Practitioner 244:785–7.

Mahoney CP. 1990. Adolescent gynecomastia. Differential diagnosis and management. Pediatr Clin North Am 37:1389–404.

Neuman JF. 1997. Evaluation and treatment of gynecomastia. Am Fam Physician 55:1835–44.

Webster DJ. 1989. Benign disorders of the male breast. World J Surg 13:726–30.

FINE-NEEDLE ASPIRATION

Oertel YC. 1987. Fine needle aspiration of the breast. Boston: Butterworths.

RADIOLOGY

Kopans DB. 1988. Breast imaging, second edition, Philadelphia: Lippincott-Raven.

Heywang-Kohbruner, Deshaw, D, Schreer I. 2001. Diagnostic breast imaging. Georg Thieme-Verlag.

Tabar L., Dean P. 1985. Teaching atlas of mammography. Georg Thieme-Verlag.

Andolini V, Lille S, Wiilison K. 1992. Mammographic imaging. Philadelphia: J.B. Lippincott.

Young W, Hoffman, N. 1994. Breast Cancer. Mt Hope Publishing Co.

PATHOLOGY

Rosen, PP. 2001. Rosen's breast pathology. Philadelphia: Lippincott Williams & Wilkins.

Tavassoli, FA. 1999. Pathology of the breast, second edition. Stamford, Conn.: Appleton & Lange.

SENTINEL NODE

Sappey PC. 1885. Anatomie, physiologie, pathologie des vesseaux lymphatiques considères chez l'homme et les vertèbres. Paris: A. Delahaye and E. Lecrosnier.

Rouvière H. 1938. Anatomie humaine, descriptive et topographique. 4th ed. Paris: Masson.

Testut L, Jacob O. 1975. Tratado de anatomia topografica. 8th ed. Barcelona: Salvat Editores.

Klinberg VS et al. 1999. Subareolar versus peritumoral injection for location of the sentinel lymph node. Ann Surg 229:860–5.

Miner TJ, Shriver CD, Flicek PR, Miner FC, Jaques DP, Maniscalco-Theberge ME, Krag DN. 1999. Guidelines for the safe use of radioactive materials during localization and resection of the sentinel lymph node. Ann Surg Oncol 6(1):75–82.

Morton DL, Wen DR, Wong JH, Economou JS, Cagle LA, Storm FK, Foshag LJ, Cochran AJ. 1992. Technical details of intraoperative lymphatic mapping for early stage melanoma. Arch Surg 127:392–9:

TECHNIQUES

Pilnik S, Steichen F. 1986. The use of the hemostatic scalpel in operation upon the breast. Surg Gynecol Obstet 162:589–91.

Thomas JG. 1882. N Y Med J 25:337.

Kraissl CJ. The selection of appropriate lines for elective surgical incision. Plastic and Reconst. Surgery. 8:1:1951.

Urban, JA. 1952. Radical mastectomy in continuity with en block resection of the internal mammary lymph node chain. Cancer 5:992.

RECONSTRUCTION

Vasconez LO, Gamboa-Bobadilla M, Lejour M. 1990. Atlas of breast reconstruction. Philadelphia: JB Lippincott; NewYork: Gower Medical.

Bostwick J 3rd. 1983. Aesthetic and reconstructive breast surgery. St. Louis: Mosby.

Hartrampf CR, Michelow BJ. 1991. Breast reconstruction with living tissue. Norfolk, VA: Hampton Press; New York: Raven Press.

Index

Abscess of breast
  consistency of lesion of, 86
  differentiated from inflammatory
    carcinoma, 41
  mastodynia in, 43, 55
  in Morgagni tubercles, 48, 48f
  nipple discharge in, 55, 55f
  skin symptoms in, 64, 78, 78f
  surgical treatment of, 184
    duct excision in, 179f, 179–180, 180f
Acini, anatomy of, 33, 136, 137
Adenoma of nipple, differentiated from
  Paget's disease, 37
Adenosis, 21, 139–140, 140f
  blunt, 21, 140, 140f, 141, 141f
  calcifications in, 21, 104, 108, 108f,
    109
    pathology in, 141, 141f
  pathology in, 139–140, 140f, 141,
    141f
  sclerosing, 21, 139–140, 140f
    calcification of, 21, 108, 108f
Adolescence, fibroadenoma in
  giant, 8–9, 9f
  juvenile, 9–10, 10f
Age, 29, 71
  in duct ectasia, 71
  in fibroadenoma, 4, 6, 71
    giant, 8–9, 111
    juvenile, 9–10
  in fibrocystic changes, 23, 71
  at first pregnancy, and breast cancer
    risk, 73
  in gynecomastia, 91–92
  in hamartoma, 10
  in lobular carcinoma in situ, 34
  in male breast carcinoma, 94
  at menarche, and breast cancer risk, 72
  at menopause, and breast cancer risk,
    72
  in nipple discharge, 50, 53, 57
  in papilloma, 71
  in phyllodes tumor, 12, 17
  in screening mammography, 101
Amastia, 79–80, 80f
Anatomy
  of areola and nipple, 47, 47f, 195
  of axilla, 82, 204f-205f, 204–205
    lymphatic, 199f-200f, 199–200, 205,
      210–211, 211f

of mammary ducts and lobules, 33,
  33f, 136–138, 137f-138f
  surgical, 195f-200f, 195–200
    in axillary lymph node dissection,
      204f-205f, 204–205
    in sentinel node dissection,
      210 211, 211f
Anesthesia
  in biopsy
    fine-needle aspiration, 167
    image-guided excisional, 186,
      187f
  in breast-conserving surgery, 200,
    201, 201f
    in re-excision, 203
    in sentinel node dissection, 213
  in duct excision, 180
  in fibroadenoma excision, 171,
    171f–172f, 175
  in gynecomastia excision, 190
Anticoagulant therapy, ecchymosis in,
  61, 61f
Apocrine cells, 139, 139f, 165, 166f
Areola
  anatomy of, 47, 47f, 195
  physical examination of, 78
    color in, 47, 78
  reconstructive surgery of, 237, 241,
    241f
Arm edema
  in axillary lymph node dissection,
    209–210
  in modified radical mastectomy, 225,
    230, 230f
  in radical mastectomy, 233
Aspiration, fine-needle, 129–130, 130f,
  165, 167–170
  advantages and disadvantages of,
    129–130
  complications of, 130, 170
  in cysts. *See* Cysts, aspiration of
  equipment used in, 168, 168f
  in fibroadenoma, 165, 166f
  indications for, 130, 167–168
  procedure in, 167, 168f-169f,
    168–170
  smear preparation in, 169–170
  ultrasound-guided, 129, 130f
Athelia, 48

Axilla
  anatomy of, 82, 204f-205f, 204–205
    lymphatic, 199f-200f, 199–200, 205,
      210–211, 211f
  extension of breast tissue to. *See*
    Axillary tail of Spence
  physical examination of, 82, 82f
Axillary artery anatomy, 205
Axillary lymph nodes
  anatomy of, 199f-200f, 199–200, 205,
    210–211, 211f
  dissection in breast-conserving
    surgery, 204–210
    closure in, 209
    complications in, 209–210
    excision technique in, 208, 208f
    historical development of, 194,
      194f-195f
    incisions in, 206f-208f, 206–208
    indications for, 205, 208–209
    level I and II, 205–208, 206f-208f
    level III, 205, 208–209, 209f
    postoperative appearance in, 209,
      209f
    of sentinel node, 210–216
    surgical technique in, 204f-209f,
      204–210
  dissection in modified radical
    mastectomy, 204, 208–209,
    222–223, 225–228
  dissection in total mastectomy, 216,
    222
  groups of, 199f, 199–200, 205
  level I
    anatomy of, 200, 200f, 205
    dissection in breast-conserving
      surgery, 205–208, 206f-208f
  level II
    anatomy of, 200, 200f, 205
    dissection in breast-conserving
      surgery, 205, 208, 208f
  level III
    anatomy of, 200, 200f, 205
    dissection in breast-conserving
      surgery, 205, 208–209, 209f
  metastasis to. *See* Metastasis to lymph
    nodes
  palpation of, 82
  sentinel. *See* Sentinel lymph node
  ultrasonography of, 118